A
Better
Understanding of
Poliomyelitis and PPS

The Central Nervous System
Poliomyelitis
The Post-poliomyelitis Syndrome

Publisher: **Tom House - Polio • Echo e. V.**
(Polio • Educational and charity help organization)

Authors: Tom House (Thomas House-Arno) and
Professor Kai Paschen MD

Contact: **Polio • Echo e. V.**
President: Tom House (Thomas House-Arno)
Weberweg 4, D-78126 Königsfeld-Buchenberg

Tel.: +49(0)7725-917604
Email: thomas.house@gmx.de

The contents of this booklet are based on excerpts from the Polio • Echo website noted below, a collection of information already distributed by Polio • Echo through electronic media means, DVDs, videos, literature and information material:

http://www.polio-echo.eu

Tom House (Thomas House-Arno) was responsible for the collection, compilation and construction of information material and facsimile with medical faculties carried out over several years with the help of Professor Kai Paschen MD. Proof reading was carried out by John McFarlane, President of the European Polio Union. This booklet is also available in German and further language versions are being pursued.

The copyrights remain with the authors. No part of this publication may be reproduced in any form without prior written permission of the publisher or duplicated using electronic systems or by any means, or disseminated.

Published in July 2015

ISBN-13: 978-1515249665
ISBN-10: 1515249662

Note: ***poliomyelitis*** *(polio) and*
Post-poliomyelitis Syndrome *(post polio syndrome)*
Those underlined definitions used in this booklet, are the official definitions declared by the WHO and Medical Convention.

Foreword by John McFarlane
(President of the European Polio Union – EPU)

As President of the EPU, I and the organisation that I represent are proud to be associated with the publication of this important document. It represents all that is best in the manner in which poliomyelitis survivors come together to form self-help groups that not only look to those closest to themselves but also in the wider poliomyelitis family across the world.

Poliomyelitis as a disease in the Western world is virtually unknown for the past 20 years but is still very much a reality in sub-Saharan Africa and in many parts of the Indian subcontinent. Whilst the eradication programme that has been ongoing for many years is an undoubted success there are still over 15 million poliomyelitis survivors around the world who will need some form of assistance and help for the rest of their lives and this will be for decades to come.

Poliomyelitis survivors are an ageing population in Europe and in North America as well as countries such as Australia. It is in these countries where the greatest knowledge regarding the management and treatment in primary care of those experiencing the Post-poliomyelitis Syndrome and Post-poliomyelitis sequelae exists. There is a very great danger that without publications such as this that knowledge will be lost to those in the greatest need in Africa and Asia. At the second Post-poliomyelitis Syndrome Conference held in Amsterdam in June 2014 the delegates were of one mind that the transference of knowledge and retention of knowledge built-up over the years in Europe is paramount. It is interesting to note, and a significant factor that the conference like its predecessor in 2011 saw a coming together of both poliomyelitis survivors and medical professionals; all dedicated to the well-being of poliomyelitis survivors wherever and whoever they are.

This publication demonstrates and illustrates best practice that allows poliomyelitis survivors to live with dignity and independence. I, and the EPU, congratulate the authors and their organisation on their hard work in adding to the body of knowledge in this field.

John R McFarlane, President European Polio Union

Foreword by Stefan Teufel MdL
(Member of the regional government of Baden-Württemberg, Germany)

Ladies and Gentlemen,

"Poliomyelitis? That doesn't exist anymore these days." This statement heard frequently, bring the challenges of an infection to light, which unfortunately receives little attention from the public nowadays.

Approximately 60,000 people in Germany suffer from the late effects of poliomyelitis (called *infantile paralysis* in earlier years). The figures show that the disease is nowhere near as meaningless as it is often portrayed. In addition to the general suffering caused by the initial poliomyelitis infection, many poliomyelitis survivors, forgotten victims of past epidemics, suffer with the so-called *Post-poliomyelitis Syndrome* many years later.

What can we do about it? In my view, a general public elucidation of this dangerous and highly contagious viral infection is extremely important. Public awareness is promoted through events such as the *World Polio Day*. The same is true for this booklet that you are holding in your hands. It shows impressively how poliomyelitis and the long-term late effects have evolved over the past number of decades and how personal counselling, the development of self-help groups and a targeted reduction of information deficits in the   population continues.

It is crucial that we all deal with the issue sensitively. We should also create a sense of acceptance for immunization in the population, making a correct and important step forward.

Yours sincerely

Stefan Teufel MdL

(Health minister spokesman of the Christian Democratic Union (CDU) of the parliamentary group Baden-Württemberg, Germany.
Chairman of the working group for social affairs of the CDU parliamentary group Baden-Württemberg, Germany)

Contents

Booklet Foreword

The majority of information regarding poliomyelitis and the Post-polio-myelitis Syndrome available on the world market is quite often expensive and sometimes difficult for the uninitiated to fully understand. The main reason for this is that it is mostly initiated and written by members of the medical profession and their usage of general professional medical scientific terminology in their explanations.

The main goal of the authors was to present this documentation using plain common language where possible, especially with the aim of making it understandable for an uninitiated poliomyelitis clientele within the wide range of existing information deficits, and further, to make this booklet obtainable at a reasonable price, therefore making it available for a wider public.

This booklet relays information about general medical basics in the relationship between a healthy human body, a human body affected by a poliomyelitis infection and its late effects. Additional graphics and illustrations underline the effort made to pursue an easier understanding of the complexity involved. It is especially helpful for poliomyelitis survivors, as well as for those who are directly involved with them such as relatives and friends, but also for nursing staff, students and physicians. If you are a poliomyelitis survivor, it should be of help for a better understanding and may be able to slow down a possible degeneration and counteract many of your problems.

Much of the information will be new for some to start with; in particular information regarding the central nervous system related to our nerve cells. You will experience some repetitions of matter that will be of great benefit to you later on in the booklet, making it easier to understand the correlations involved when the impact of the polio-myelitis virus on our human system and the late effects, the Post-poliomyelitis Syndrome, are explained.

Without the global work of self-help organizations, many poliomyelitis survivors will continue to go from one doctor to another and may never really get to know that the cause of their symptoms is related to the original poliomyelitis infection. They may be falsely or not properly diagnosed and perhaps advised for wrong treatment. In many cases, some uninformed doctors may even refer to them as being malingerers.

Introduction

Poliomyelitis, also known as infantile paralysis, is caused by a highly infectious virus. Poliomyelitis can be potentially fatal. On infection, the poliomyelitis virus generally attacks the motor nerve cells (*alpha motor neurons*), particularly those in the spinal cord that carry messages (*electrical impulses*) between the spinal cord and the muscles in order for them to function and can cause severe muscle paralysis (*paralytic poliomyelitis*), including severe damage to nerve cells in several control centres of the brain.

Firstly, we should know a little bit about how our central nervous system (CNS) functions in order to understand the impact regarding the immediate consequences of a poliomyelitis infection and the PPS.

Here are some photographs of poliomyelitis survivors of then and now:

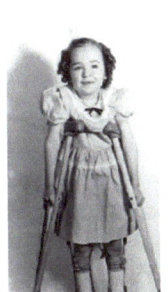 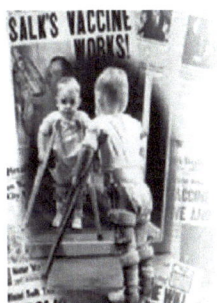 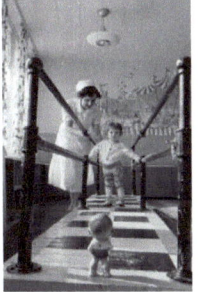 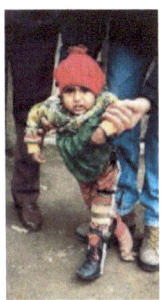

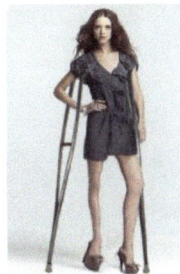 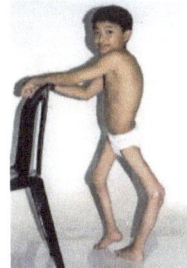 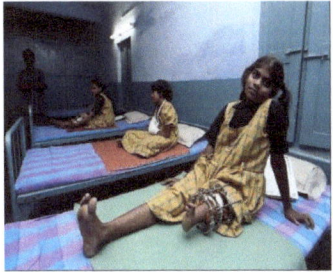

The Central Nervous System (CNS)

The CNS controls the functions of vital organs of the body including functions of movement and senses: −> thinking, feeling and action. It is responsible for processing the complex network of nerves to ensure that the organs work correctly. The CNS interprets-, stores- and responds to information received from the outside environment and within the body.

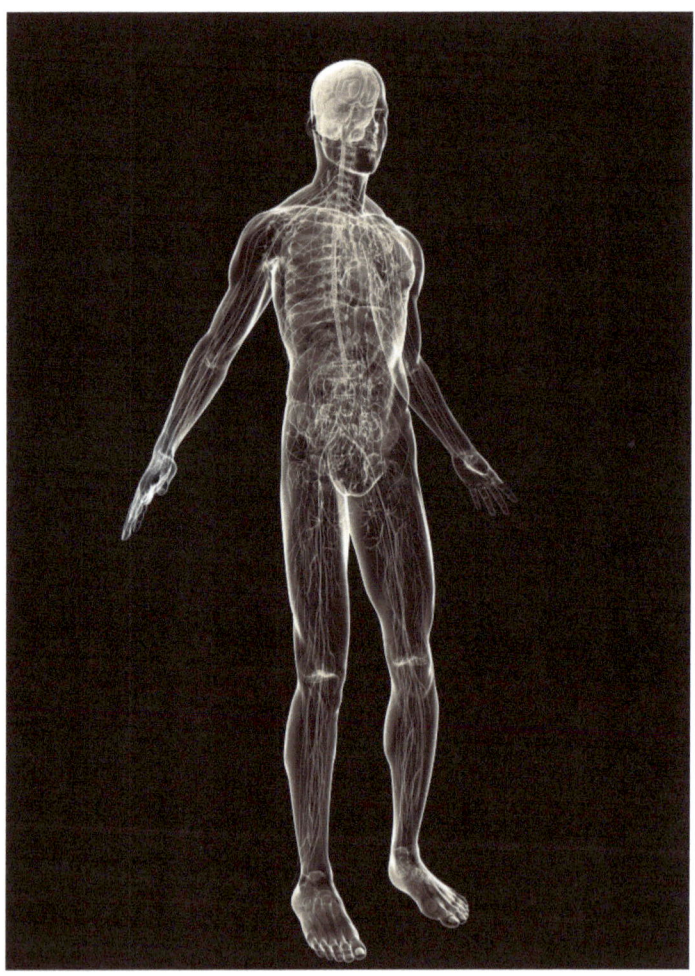

Brain and Spinal Cord

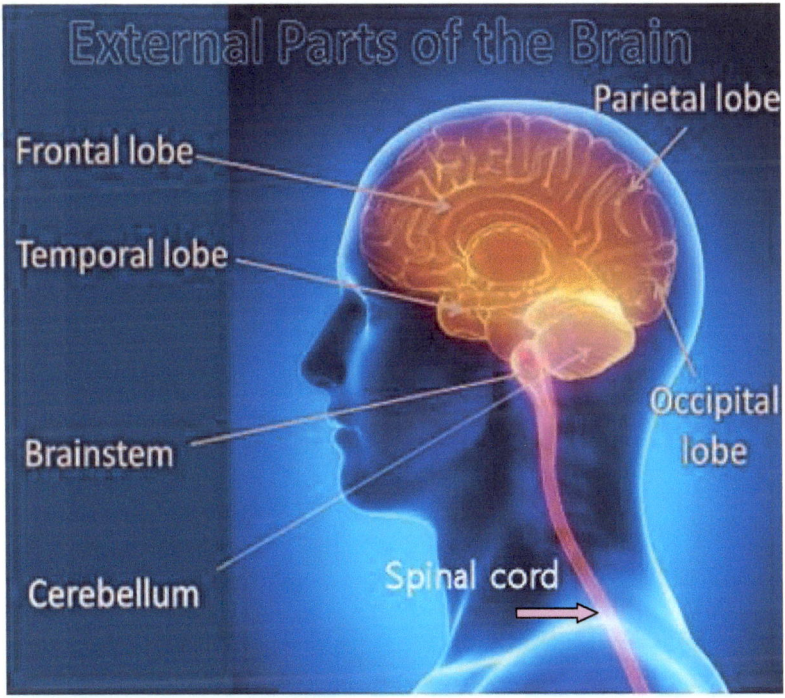

Our brain weighs approximately 1300 grams and requires a quarter of the available body energy in order to supply more than 100 billion nerve cells. The cells are connected to each other by more than 100 trillion transmitters (synapses). This allows the brain to process up to 750 million pulses per second. The brain is thus able to send more than 450 million signals per second, for example, to the muscles.

Nerve Cell and Nerve String

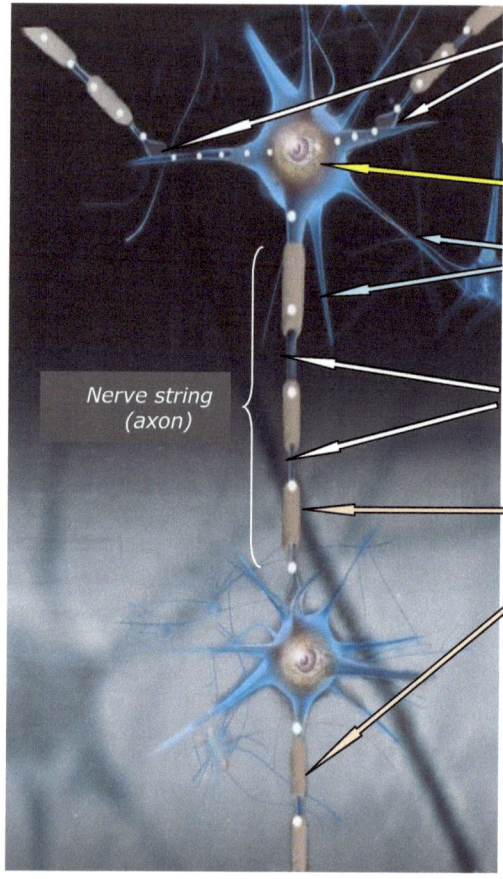

Synaptic end nodes
Nerve cell terminal:
Docking place for signals
from other nerve cells.

Cell core (Nerve control
centre)

Signal receiving nodes
(*Dendrites*)

Ranvier nodes

Mark sheath
Insulating layers ->
(Myelin sheath) =
Nerve string protection
layer

*Nerve string
(axon)*

The nerve string (*axon*). The receiving nodes (dendrites) receive impulse signals from other nerve cells. The control centre of the receiving nerve cell relays the impulses to further nerve cells via its nerve string. The nerve string is protected by insulating layers called Mark sheaths (*Myelin sheaths*) that guarantee fast transportation of the electrical impulses. The Mark sheaths are separated by Ranvier nodes that enable a constant and accelerated transportation of the impulses through the nerve string.

The Mark sheath (Myelin sheath) is made up of several fatty insulation layers. The myelin sheath is regularly constricted by Ranvier nodes, at which points the nerve cord membrane is freed. The nerve strings terminate in synaptic end nodes of other nerve cells (***intermediary bodies***). This means that an extensive exchange of communication between nerve cells takes place that are controlled by electrical and chemical processes. The nerve cells are designed to receive stimuli (signal impulses) and transmit impulses to other nerve cells. The end *terminal* of the nerve string has sprouted fibres that innervate specific muscle fibres.

Brain and spinal cord form the central nervous system (CNS). Its function is to interpret, store and respond to information received from the environment outside and inside the body. The spinal cord begins directly under the brain stem (medulla oblongata), the lower portion of the brain. The 12 so-called cranial nerves originate directly from the brain and not from the spinal cord. They provide the main motor and sensory innervation to the eyes, nose, face, ears, neck and small parts of the upper shoulder belt.

The spinal cord provides the connection between the brain and the peripheral nervous system (PNS). Depending on gender and body size, the spinal cord is approximately 45 cm long and has 31 pairs of spinal nerves that branch off the spinal cord through inter-vertebral foramen.

Spinal Cord

The spinal cord is a prolonged extension of the brain that is surrounded by fluid and closed in by skin layers similar to the meningeal.

The spinal cord is of cylindrical shape and consists of a white and gray matter.

The **gray matter** in the centre of the spinal cord, is shaped like a butterfly and consists of cell bodies of inter-neurons and motor neurons. Projections of the gray matter (wings) are called horns.

The **white matter** is located outside of the gray matter and consists mostly of myelinated axons that serve as long pathways to and from the brain to the neurons within the spinal cord.

The axons of sensory neurons (afferent sensory axons) *ENTER* the posterior horn (dorsal horn), whereas the axons of the motor neurons *LEAVE* the spinal cord via the anterior horn.

All conductive paths join in the so-called spinal ganglion to form a nerve serving a specific part of the body. The spinal cord is closed in and protected by various skin layers similar to the meningeal. The brain-spinal fluid (liquor cerebrospinalis) flows between the skin layers and the medulla.

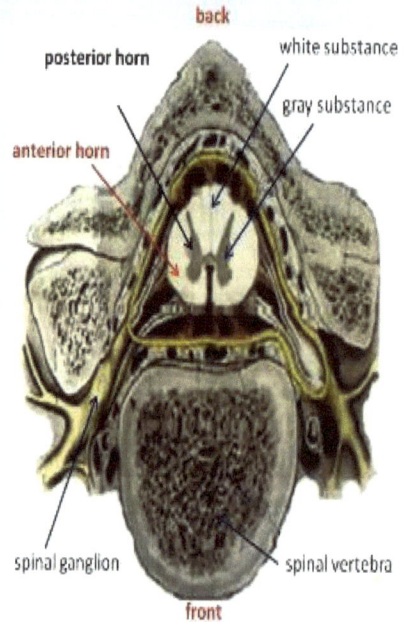

back

posterior horn

white substance

gray substance

anterior horn

spinal ganglion

spinal vertebra

front

Spinal ganglia. Each segment of the spinal cord is associated with a pair of ganglia called dorsal root ganglia (accumulation of nerve cells) that are situated on the exterior of the spinal cord and contain cell bodies of sensory nerve cells (from afferent sensory nerve strings), picked up by sensory receptors throughout the body (PNS) and carried *TOWARDS* the spinal cord + brain (CNS).

Ventral roots. These consist of nerve strings of motor nerve cells (alpha motor neurons) of the anterior horn, as well as, in some spinal cord sections, fibres of the autonomic nervous system (ANS – see page 20). Their cell bodies are situated in the central part of the gray substance and transport information to the periphery from cell bodies within the CNS. The nerve strings of motor nerve cells (efferent) are assembled AWAY from the CNS through the spinal ganglion to form nerves of the PNS that innervate the specific body muscles. The nerve strings of motor nerve cells innervate striated *muscle fibres*, simply referred to as *muscle fibres* that are located throughout the muscle.

Of the more than 100 billion nerve cells in our body, we shall generally concentrate on the motor nerve cells in this booklet. Motor nerve cells are responsible for the management of our skeletal muscle system and are prone to attack and destruction by the poliomyelitis virus.

(Let's recapitulate what we have just learnt !)

Each motor nerve cell consists of three main components - the cell body (control centre), numerous signal receiving nodes (small branching fibres = dendrites) and the main nerve string (axon).

The nerve cells are designed to receive stimuli (signal impulses) and transmit impulses to other nerve cells. The nerve strings terminate in synaptic end nodes of other nerve cells (***intermediary bodies***). This means that an extensive exchange of communication between nerve cells takes place that are controlled by electrical and chemical processes.

The end ***terminal*** of the nerve string has sprouted fibres that innervate specific muscle fibres.

Motor Nerve Cell - Communication Course

The signal receiving nodes of the motor nerve cell receive stimuli from other motor nerve cells and the nerve string relays (passes on) the stimuli to other motor nerve cells, the motor endplate of the muscle fibre, or other organ. The nerve strings are protected by insulating layers called Mark sheaths that guarantee coordinated fast transportation of the electrical impulses. The Mark sheaths are separated by Ranvier nodes that enable a regular constricted and accelerated transportation of the impulses through to the end point of the nerve string (synaptic end nodes - intermediary points = synapses). At this point the nerve string terminates and the nerve cord membrane is freed and the impulse passed on chemically over a hair-thin gap to another motor nerve cell (intermediary body), motor endplate of the muscle fibre or other organ, using so-called nerve transmitters (neuro transmitters). This means that an extensive exchange of communication between nerve cells takes place that are controlled by electrical and chemical processes. The nerve cells are designed to receive stimuli (signal impulses) and transmit these to other nerve cells.

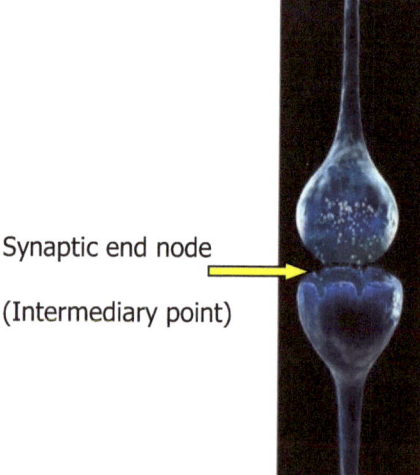

Synaptic end node

(Intermediary point)

Several nerve strings and their Mark sheaths form nerve fibres. There are sensory, motor- and autonomic nerve fibres. Sensory fibres conduct stimuli of specific sensory organs (eye, ear, tongue). Motor nerve fibres supply the muscles. The autonomic fibres are nerves of the vegetative (autonomous) nervous system. Nerve cell information of all organisms is passed on via electrical currents.

Here is a simple illustration of three healthy motor nerve cells with their corresponding nerve strings and the sprouted fibres of the end terminals that innervate and serve some upper-arm muscle fibres.

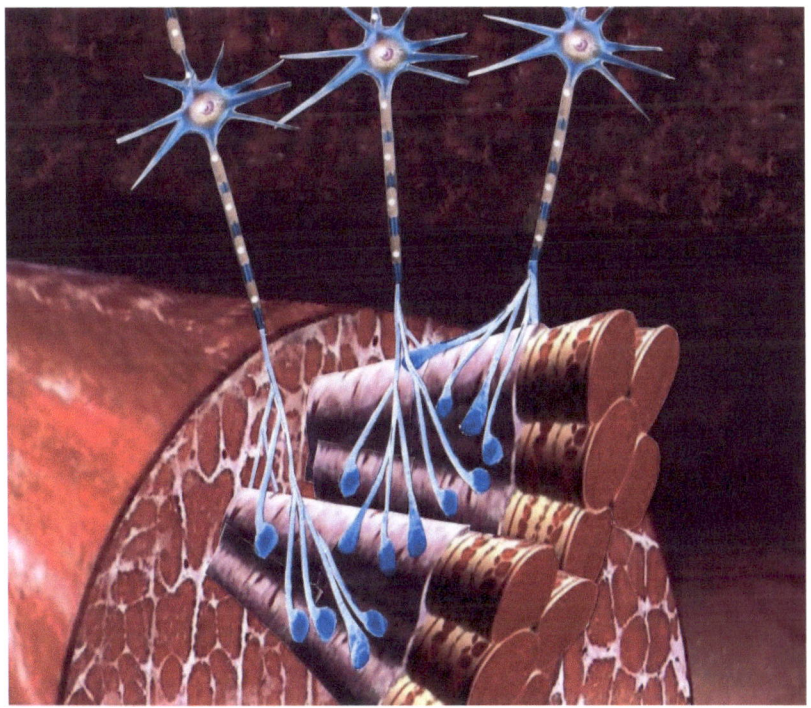

The nerve strings from the anterior horn of the spinal cord transmit the nerve impulses of those particular nerve strings to the appropriate muscle fibres. A muscle is composed of many muscle fibre bundles. Muscles are machines that transform chemical energy directly into mechanical energy and heat.

The above illustration shows a section of a striated skeletal muscle in an upper arm, made up of several muscle fibre bundles bound together by connective tissue and attached to a bone by collagen bundles called tendons. Skeletal muscles are attached to the bone and are moved by contraction. This is initiated by nerve impulses under voluntary control. The active elements of muscle cells are the filaments of the protein bodies: myosin and actin. Having the relevant appropriate nerve impulses, the actin filaments slide into the myosin filaments and thus ensure the contraction of the muscle.

Structure of the Central Nervous System (CNS)

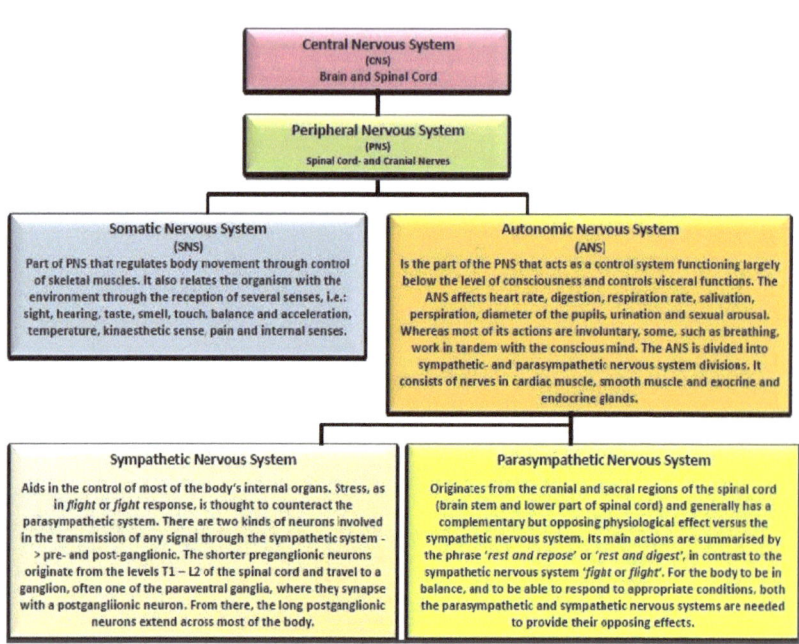

Central Nervous System
(CNS)
Brain and Spinal Cord

Peripheral Nervous System
(PNS)
Spinal Cord- and Cranial Nerves

Somatic Nervous System
(SNS)
Part of PNS that regulates body movement through control of skeletal muscles. It also relates the organism with the environment through the reception of several senses, i.e.: sight, hearing, taste, smell, touch, balance and acceleration, temperature, kinaesthetic sense, pain and internal senses.

Autonomic Nervous System
(ANS)
Is the part of the PNS that acts as a control system functioning largely below the level of consciousness and controls visceral functions. The ANS affects heart rate, digestion, respiration rate, salivation, perspiration, diameter of the pupils, urination and sexual arousal. Whereas most of its actions are involuntary, some, such as breathing, work in tandem with the conscious mind. The ANS is divided into sympathetic- and parasympathetic nervous system divisions. It consists of nerves in cardiac muscle, smooth muscle and exocrine and endocrine glands.

Sympathetic Nervous System
Aids in the control of most of the body's internal organs. Stress, as in *flight* or *fight* response, is thought to counteract the parasympathetic system. There are two kinds of neurons involved in the transmission of any signal through the sympathetic system -> pre- and post-ganglionic. The shorter preganglionic neurons originate from the levels T1 – L2 of the spinal cord and travel to a ganglion, often one of the paraventral ganglia, where they synapse with a postganglionic neuron. From there, the long postganglionic neurons extend across most of the body.

Parasympathetic Nervous System
Originates from the cranial and sacral regions of the spinal cord (brain stem and lower part of spinal cord) and generally has a complementary but opposing physiological effect versus the sympathetic nervous system. Its main actions are summarised by the phrase *'rest and repose'* or *'rest and digest'*, in contrast to the sympathetic nervous system *'fight* or *flight'*. For the body to be in balance, and to be able to respond to appropriate conditions, both the parasympathetic and sympathetic nervous systems are needed to provide their opposing effects.

Communication is the basis of human existence. One not only communicates with the environment, but also with one's inner world, with one's body. Body cells communicate with each other.

The complex network of the central nervous system consists of the

Brain and Spinal Cord.

The rest of the body is controlled by the peripheral nervous system, a network of nerves that transmits signals through the spinal cord between the brain and muscles, skin and body organs. They are in constant contact and control any conscious or random movement and action of striated skeletal muscles, and the unconscious or involuntary movements in smooth muscles, such as the control of digestion and heart.

The **peripheral nervous system** is divided into two sub-parts. One group of nerves – the **somatic nerves** that are connected to the muscles of the body, inter alia, can be controlled consciously or arbitrarily. For example, if one wants to move the big toe, this system works jointly with the brain and spinal cord in order to implement the desire for action. The other group of nerves – the **autonomic or vegetative nerves** – are connected to the unconscious or involuntarily controlled operating regions, e.g. the salivary glands and digestive visceral muscles (visceral = internal organs). These nerves control involuntary body functions to maintain a constant internal state. They regulate, e.g. blood pressure and body temperature.

The **vegetative (autonomic) nervous system** in turn is divided into the **sympathetic** and **parasympathetic nervous system** - also called the **vagus**:

> The **sympathetic nervous system** starts from the spinal cord, forming a chain of ganglia (clusters of nerve cell bodies, including the corresponding nerve strings) that run up the spine. The SNS prepares the body for activity and energy consumption. This nerve group, inter alia, increases the heart rate and blood pressure and leads to dilation of the pupils.

> The **parasympathetic nervous system** starts from the upper (cranial) and lower (sacral) end of the nervous system and relaxes the body to restore energy. It acts, e.g. on the facial nerve that controls the secretion of saliva and tear glands, and the digestive tract (stomach/intestine).

Poliomyelitis – Illness

Poliomyelitis is a viral infection of the intestinal virus family (Enterovirus) that spread quickly through the body, attacking muscles and tissue of the central nervous system.

Initially, the poliomyelitis virus multiplies in lymphoid tissues (tonsils and intestinal lymph nodes) and then quickly spreads through the bloodstreams (hematogenously) throughout the body.

As a so-called nerve-type virus (neuro-tropic), it attacks motor nerve cells of the brain and spinal cord (alpha motor nerve cells) and is excreted orally or in the stool.

It destroys some of the motor nerve cells (alpha motor neurons) and the corresponding nerve strings (axons). The corresponding muscle fibres lose contact and are no longer innervated. This results in a flaccid paralysis.

Many motor nerve cells are now destroyed or irreparably damaged. During the recovery phase, surviving motor nerve cells serving the same muscle sprout new fibres to innervate some of the orphaned striated muscle fibres that were previously innervated by the dead nerve cells.

While this promotes a certain recovery of muscles, it places additional stress on the nerve cell body to nourish the additional fibres. The survived motor cell nerves enlarge, now having to support more muscle fibres. These are called giant motor units. This is a repairing mechanism that occurs after the acute poliomyelitis phase to support paralysed muscle groups.

Poliomyelitis causes brain damage. According to current findings, the poliomyelitis infection not only affects the peripheral nervous system but the brain as well. Therefore, it is not only a peripheral muscular nerve illness. Of more clinical importance is often possible damage to the brain – the encephalic portion (e.g. respiration -> whereby the patient has to be placed in an 'iron lung', etc.).

Poliomyelitis – Course of Infection

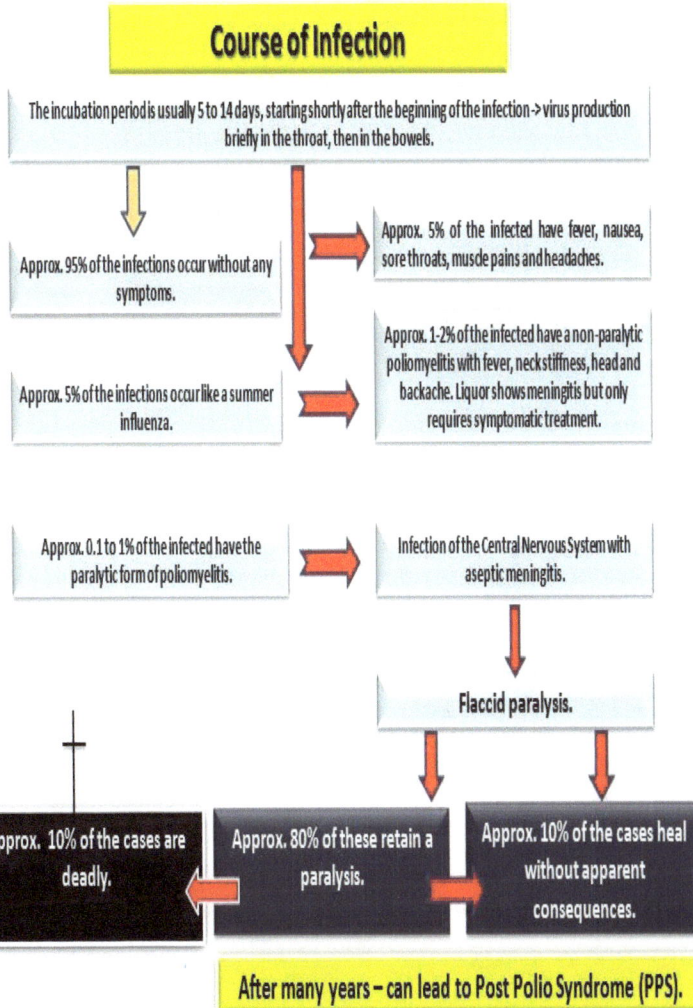

Poliomyelitis – Primary Damage

Poliomyelitis means cerebral (brain) and spinal cord inflammation and used to be called infantile paralysis because at the time doctors thought that only children caught the disease.

When the poliomyelitis virus infects the body, it affects nerve cells in the control centre called motor nerve cells (motor neurons), particularly those in the spinal cord (alpha motor neurons) that carry messages (electrical impulses) between the brain and the skeletal muscles. A poliomyelitis infection leaves many of these motor nerve cells destroyed or damaged.

An infection by the poliomyelitis virus can cause the following damage or symptoms:

* Severe nerve damage (brain and skeletal muscles),
* Paralyses, loose and floppy limbs (flaccid paralysis),
* Severe pain, back, neck and extremities,
* Touch sensitivity(sensitivity afferences),
* Encephalo meningitis,
* Difficulty breathing –> iron lung,
* or even

death.

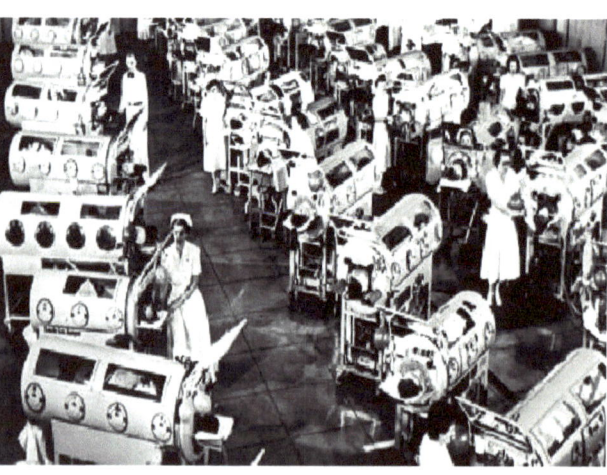

Iron
Lungs

If poliomyelitis is treated correctly in the early stages of the infection, this may minimize the severe after effects that may occur and may also help to save the life of some patients who may otherwise die during the acute stage.

Poliomyelitis Survivors

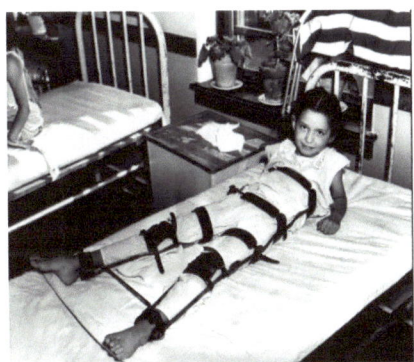
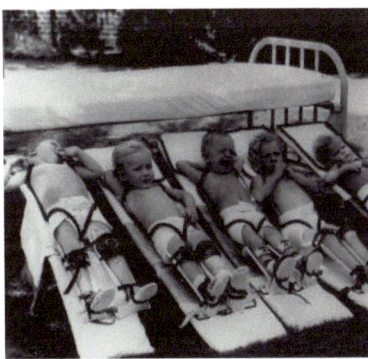

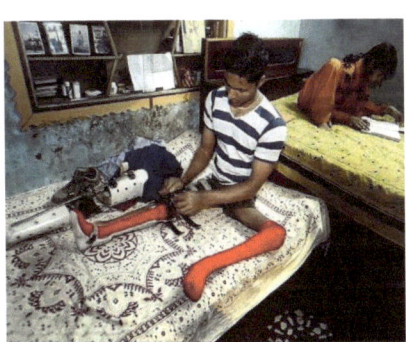
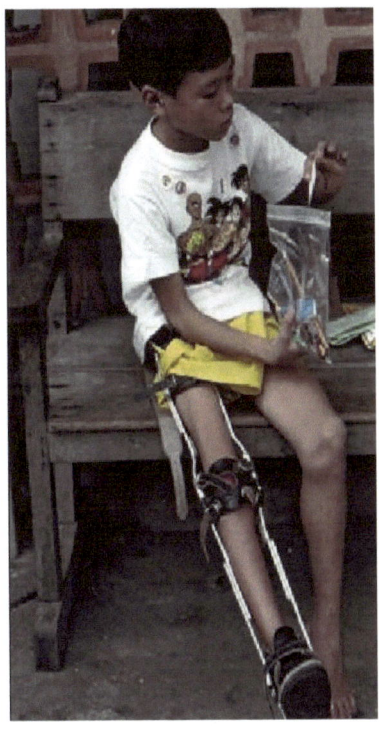

Poliomyelitis – Symptoms & Diagnosis

In ca. 95% of acute poliomyelitis virus infections no symptoms show, although according to recent findings there are always certain damages that do occur.

In a coverage area of less than about 50% of damaged nerve cells, no symptoms occur at all. This is because other neighbouring nerve cells take over the work of the dead cells => (plasticity of the nervous system).

In about 5% of infections, influenza-like symptoms (non-paralytic poliomyelitis) occur only for a few days.

Only in about 0.1% to 1% of cases, the infection results in a more or less pronounced flaccid paralysis (paralytic poliomyelitis), in some cases even death.

In the latter two cases, the following symptoms that occur in a period of between 1 to 10 days are important for the diagnosis:

Fever
Sore throat
Headache
Fatigue
Back pain or stiffness
Neck pain or stiffness
Pain or stiffness in the arms or legs
Muscle spasms or sensitivity/tenderness feeling
Meningitis

In addition, the following symptoms are usually observed on a polio-myelitis infection:

Loss of reflexes
Muscle pains
Flaccid paralysis, usually in different degrees

Following some, or all of the symptoms, the diagnosis is made after a thorough medical examination and assessment of the person's medical history. For an accurate diagnosis, the poliomyelitis must be differentiated from all fever type (febrile) infections caused by other agents (pathogens). The following illnesses and conditions that have similar symptoms to poliomyelitis have to be taken into consideration by the MD/physician:

-   Meningitis symptoms that occur with paralyses can also be caused by other agents from the group of intestinal viruses.

-   During the course of the brainstem (bulbar) form, Diphtheria, which has becomes rare, plays an important part in the differential diagnosis.

-   In contrast to poliomyelitis, the *Guillain Barré* syndrome, characterized by continuously ascending paralyses symmetrically from the feet, fever and a stiff neck; indications of meningitis are missing.

-   Neuro borreliosis after a tick bite.

Laboratory Analysis

Direct virus detection:

Evidence was extremely time consuming and expensive up to 1990 (cell culture growth and differentiation through neutralization tests with specific antiserum), therefore inadequate for virological routine diagnostics. In most cases the diagnosis was based on the clinical picture.

Nowadays the reverse transcriptase polymerase chain reaction (RT-PCR) is mainly used, in which the viral RNA (ribonucleic acid) in the patient sample (stool samples, throat swabs or spinal fluid) can be directly detected. Even the viral genetic material (genome) to establish a connection between different people through so-called sequence alignments can be determined. This makes it possible to trace routes of infection – also to distinguish the respective type (Type 1, 2 or 3), or wild virus from the vaccine virus or its genetically modified mutants.

According to the law in most countries, a proven poliomyelitis virus infection has to be notified to the health authorities of the particular country.

Indirect virus detection

Nowadays, determination of antibodies is rarely carried out with the poliomyelitis virus. Laboratory diagnosis of a previously experienced poliomyelitis infection is still not possible with reasonable assurance, as to-date there are no laboratory-grade-tests that can distinguish between antibodies of the wild virus from the vaccine viruses produced by induced antibodies. Antibody *Titre* determining is likewise unsuitable.

The study of cerebral spinal fluid mostly shows appropriate typical findings in an accompanying encephalitis or meningitis.

Poliomyelitis Therapy in the Acute Stage

A poliomyelitis infection cannot be cured. Therefore, the focus is on the treatment of poliomyelitis patients during the acute stage, for them to gain a rapid recovery of physical strength in order to avoid unnecessary complications from the infection.

Main important factors for the treatment are:

- Complete bed rest (2-3 weeks)

- Good whole-food nutrition

- Early start with mild passive physical therapy

- Intensive skin care and special bed-laying positions to prevent bedsores (decubitus), or contractures.

- If necessary, mechanical breathing support

- Possible pain treatment

After the acute therapy, it is extremely important for all poliomyelitis patients, especially those infected with the paralytic form, to carry on with physical therapy treatment.

Poliomyelitis – What Happens After That?

In the illustration below is an example of healthy nerve strings before the infection: 3 nerve cells with their nerve strings and end sprouts, that supply (innervate) upper arm muscle fibres:

Healthy nerve strings (axons)

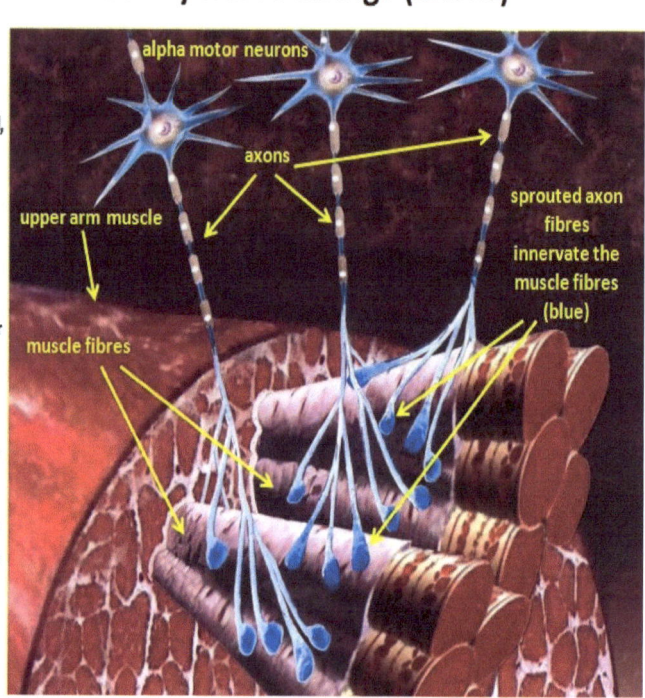

Signals for determined, i.e. arbitrary muscle movement are transported through motor neurons.

Their associated long nerve strings (axons) are bundled with other axons and

run from the spinal cord to the muscle fibres of the particular musculature.

The sprouted fibres of the axon innervate the muscle fibres.

The poliomyelitis virus may not only destroy a number of control centres in the brain (e. g. respiratory centre, circulatory centre, sleep-/rhythmic centre, temperature centre, etc.), it also destroys many motor control cells in the spinal cord responsible for the skeletal muscles and their respective nerve strings, causing a flaccid paralyses. The loss of the motor nerve cells and their nerve strings means that the corresponding muscle fibres lose contact and are no longer innervated. Many of the motor nerve cells are completely   destroyed or irreparably damaged.

Here is the same illustration example as before, showing the same nerve cells and strings but this time they are infected by the poliomyelitis virus:

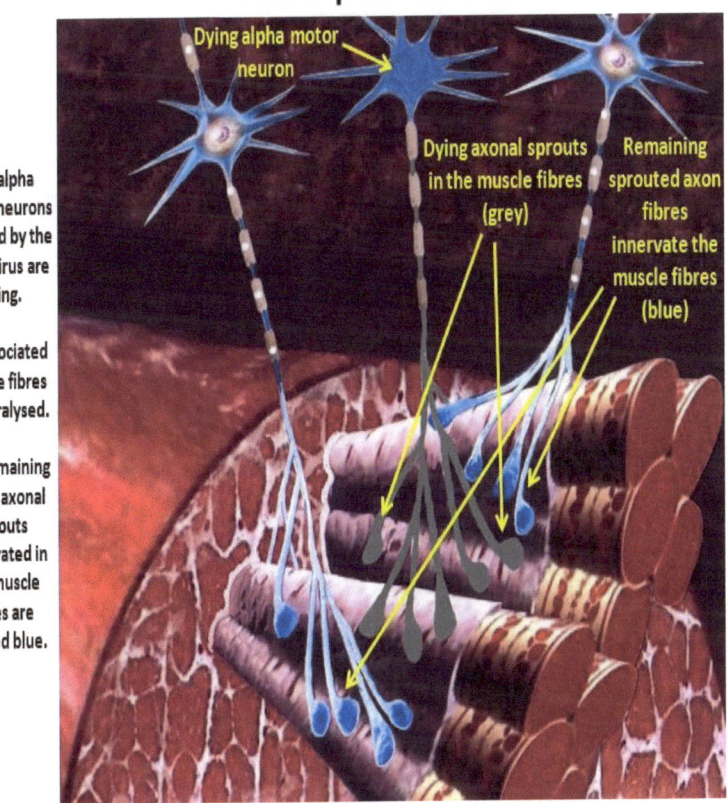

Acute polio infection

After the illness and during the recovery phase, surviving motor nerve cells (neurons) serving the same muscle sprout new fibres to innervate some of the orphaned muscle fibres that were previously innervated by the destroyed nerve cells and their nerve strings (axons). This happens during the rehabilitation phase and when physical treatment is applied – a slow muscle build-up period.

Recuperation phase after the infection

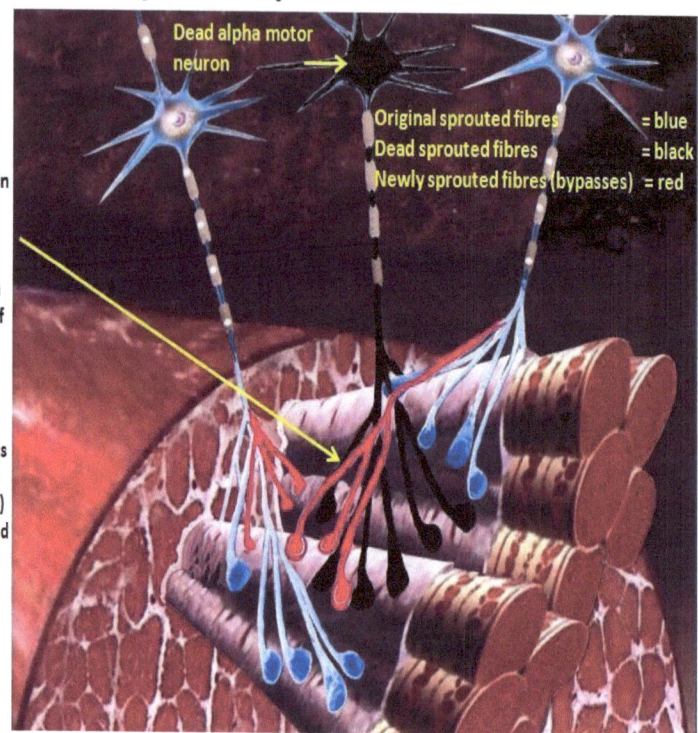

Newly sprouted axonal fibres in red.

This means that axons in the vicinity of the dead axon(s) develop additional axonal sprouts to innervate (compensate) the abandoned (destroyed) axonal sprouted fibres.

Dead alpha motor neuron

Original sprouted fibres = blue
Dead sprouted fibres = black
Newly sprouted fibres (bypasses) = red

While this promotes a certain recovery of muscles, it places additional stress on the nerve cell to nourish the additional fibres. The survived motor nerve cells enlarge, having to support more muscle fibres. These enlarge to form giant motor units. This is a repairing mechanism that occurs after the acute poliomyelitis phase to support paralysed muscle groups.

Compensation – Re-modelling

Re-modelling means that motor neurons, which formed new bypasses in the recovery phase, now serve many more (multiple) muscle fibres than before.
This is defined as a giant motor unit.

This adjustment is not static, meaning old bypasses are being constantly replaced by the regeneration of new ones.

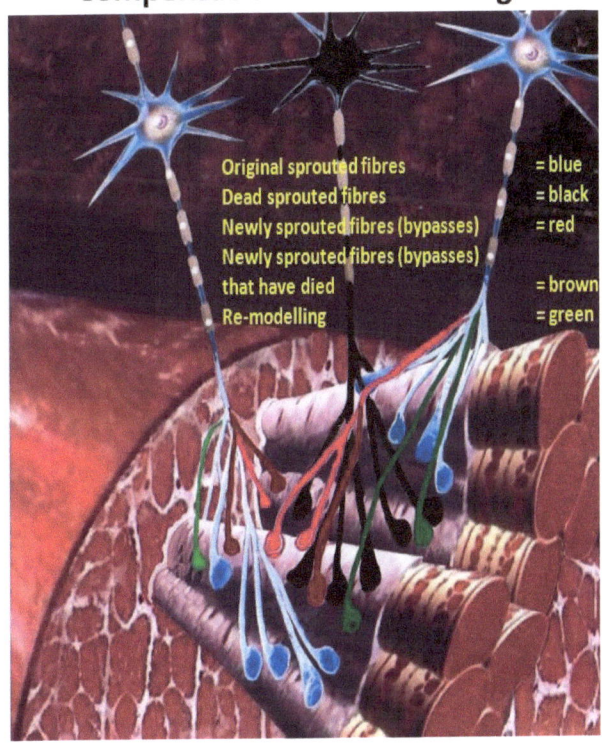

Original sprouted fibres   = blue
Dead sprouted fibres   = black
Newly sprouted fibres (bypasses)   = red
Newly sprouted fibres (bypasses)
that have died   = brown
Re-modelling   = green

Compensation – Re-modelling

This means that muscle cells thicken through regular training after the recovery phase and become more powerful. The two compensatory mechanisms: muscle growth and improving the nerve supply by increasing new nerve string sprouting, are very effective. Half of the motor nerve cells can be lost without the normal muscle strength being clinically noted as having decreased. However, these adjustments are neither static nor permanent. After recovery from the acute infection, the motor units are re-modelled continuously:

Old synaptic contacts diminish, at the same time, new ones are created.

These dynamics of permanent repair are based on a purely external constant power output. If the balance between dismantling and reassembly is disturbed, this may lead to renewed weakness.

Some poliomyelitis patients may have to remain in wheelchairs, or wear orthotics, etc. after the acute phase. Others may be lucky and be able to physically achieve more than before the infection. However, it is now known and generally accepted by medical experts, that owing to the re-generation (build-up of the giant motor units), many poliomyelitis survivors continuously stretch their physical limits to the utmost. After a period of 15-40 years, this results in a degeneration of the giant motor units, finally ending with the Post-poliomyelitis Syndrome.

What we learn from that is – **yes, to muscle build-up in the initial phase** after the illness, **but never going beyond the limits during the years after.**

This may be helpful in keeping PPS at bay.

Risks of Catching a Poliomyelitis Infection

The poliomyelitis virus affects humans and anthropoid apes (Orang-Utans, Gorillas und Chimpanzees), the only well-known carriers. The infection is through faecal-oral contact, but also from droplet infection (coughing, sneezing) from a person or anthropoid ape infected by the virus. Therefore being in the following places mean a great risk of catching a poliomyelitis infection:

- Being in areas with poor sanitation (on holiday, business trips, etc.), or

- being in areas where the vaccine is either not given, or is only given sporadically (under-developed countries, war-torn areas, etc.), or

- pregnant, or

- being so young that the immune system is not fully developed, or

- having a congenital or acquired immune deficiency (taking immune suppressants after organ transplantation, cytostatic therapy for malignant diseases, etc.), or

- residing in poliomyelitis endemic regions, or

- having had close contact with persons from endemic areas (refugees, war-wounded, etc.), or

- treating poliomyelitis patients (doctors, nurses), or

- in close contact with people from medical laboratories carrying out studies with poliomyelitis viruses, or even working there.

The Poliomyelitis Virus

The poliomyelitis virus is a micro virus (*Picorna viridae*), of the intestinal virus type (*Entero viridae*). The virus quickly spreads through the body within hours or days and can cause paralyses.

It is structurally similar to the human intestinal virus.

This is a very simple virus without casing with a genotype of single-plus-RNA (ribonucleic acid). Other well-known types are the Coxsackie A + B viruses or the ECHO virus. There are three extremely infectious types of the poliomyelitis virus:

- **Serum type 1 (**Mahoney or Brunhilde)

  This type occurs most often – the cause of epidemics and grave illness.

- **Serum type 2** (Lansing)

  This type has a mild course.

- **Serum type 3** (Leon)

  This type is seldom but the course is generally severe. Wild types are found in Nigeria, Niger, Pakistan and Sudan.

Due to its structure, the poliomyelitis virus is an environmentally stable virus, resistant to many commonly used disinfectants such as 70% ethanol, Isopropanol and quarternary ammonium base. Even with the use of detergents or acids, e.g. gastric acid, the virus can hardly be inactivated.

The poliomyelitis virus needs a specific receptor to cause an infection: – the CD155 protein on the host cells: monocytes, macrophages, T-lymphocytes and nerve cells. Reproduction takes place in the cytoplasm of the host cell. The virus is spread by smear infection (oral faeces) and via objects. After the virus has been absorbed in the mouth and the reproduction has taken place in both the lymphatic tissue of the nasopharyngeal cavity and in the digestive tract, a virus infection (virämia) occurs causing the virus to be distributed via the bloodstream.

Proof of a poliomyelitis virus infection can be made through tests on faeces samples, throat swab samples and brain-spinal fluid (liquor cerebrospinalis). Nowadays, it is carried out by means of the so-called RT-PCR, whereby viral RNA can be proven. Only parts of the virus genome need be sequenced. The then sequenced material, humans to humans, can be compared to determine the infection path. A proof of anti-bodies against the virus can also be accomplished through the patient's serum.

According to the WHO and European law, it is compulsory to notify health authorities of a positive proof of a poliomyelitis virus infection.

Epidemics occurred from about 1880. Originally, the virus was spread throughout the world. In the tropics epidemics occurred throughout the year – in temperate latitudes, especially in summer. The virus can be detected in waste water, inter alia, of epidemic areas. It is capable of reproduction in the environment for several weeks. The virus is currently endemic mainly in Africa (broad belt from the Gold Coast to Somalia and in South Africa), as well as in Pakistan and Afghanistan (constantly clustering of cases in a limited area or population).

Vaccination against Poliomyelitis

In Europe and most other countries, all children and adults should be vaccinated against poliomyelitis according to the guidelines of the Government or Committee Authorities responsible for Vaccination in their respective country. If anyone is unsure of being fully vaccinated, then their respective doctor/GP should be consulted.

The Vaccine
For Young Children

Poliomyelitis vaccine is normally part of the combined DTaP/IPV (poliomyelitis)/Hib injection – this stands for 'diphtheria, tetanus, pertussis = (whooping cough), poliomyelitis and Haemophilus influenzae type b', which is given as part of the routine childhood immunisation program.

For Teenagers and Adults

For adults and teenagers who are to receive poliomyelitis immunisation, the combined Td/IPV (poliomyelitis) vaccine is normally used. This stands for 'tetanus, diphtheria and poliomyelitis'.

The Vaccine stimulates the body to build antibodies against the poliomyelitis virus. These antibodies give protection from the poliomyelitis illness should a person come in contact with this virus.

It is safe to be given if pregnant or breast feeding.

Prior to 1989, the polio vaccine was given as drops into the mouth. It is now always given as an injection. If you have previously started a course of polio immunisation with oral vaccine you can finish off the course with polio injections. You do not need to start again.

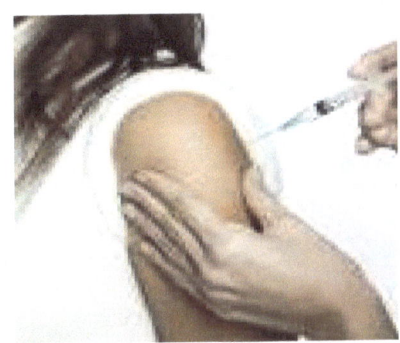

Poliomyelitis Immunisation Timetable

All children are offered poliomyelitis immunisation as part of the routine immunisation program. A full course of poliomyelitis immunisation consists of five doses of vaccine as follows:

Children	
Primary course	Three doses of vaccine – as DTaP/IPV (poliomyelitis)/Hib at two, three and four months of age.
4th dose	Three years after primary course – as part of the DTaP/IPV (poliomyelitis) pre-school refresher at 3 years and four months to 5 years.
5th dose	Aged 13-18 years – the school leaver refresher – as Td/IPV (poliomyelitis).
Adults **(who have not been immunised as a child)**	
Primary course	Three doses of vaccine – as Td/IPV (poliomyelitis), each one month apart.
4th dose	Five years after primary course – as Td/IPV (poliomyelitis).
5th dose	Ten years after 4th dose as Td/IPV(poliomyelitis).

The primary course of three injections gives good protection for a number of years. The fourth and fifth doses (refresher) are needed in later years to maintain protection. After the fifth dose, immunity remains for life and further refreshers (apart from some travel situations – see *Travellers* below) are not needed.

Indications for the Poliomyelitis Vaccination of Adults

Unvaccinated persons receive IPV (inactivated poliomyelitis vaccine) according to the manufacturer.
Pending (incomplete) vaccinations of the primary series can be caught-up with an IPV vaccination refresher. A routine refresher is not recommended after the age of 18.
Members of the following groups should possess recent poliomyelitis vaccination immunity. *(Refresh the poliomyelitis vaccination immunity by IPV if the last vaccine dose was given more than 10 years ago, otherwise primary vaccination or completion of missing vaccinations)*:

- **All persons who do not have an immunization or who only have an incomplete basic immunization.**
- **All persons without at least one refresher.**
- **For the following categories of persons a refresher vaccination is indicated:**
  - **Travellers in regions with risk of infection (the current epidemic situation is to be observed, in particular WHO reports).**
  - **Emigrants, refugees and asylum seekers living in collective living quarters, coming from areas with poliomyelitis risk.**
  - **Staff of the previously mentioned institutions.**
  - **Medical personnel in close contact with polio-myelitis infected patients.**
  - **Staff in laboratories with poliomyelitis risk.**
  - **On a poliomyelitis infection, all contact persons should receive vaccination with IPV without delay, regardless of vaccination status.**
  - **A secondary case is cause for a regular vaccination with IPV.**

Side-effects of the Poliomyelitis Vaccine

- Slight swelling and redness at the injection site is common.
- A little area of hard skin may form at the injection site, which usually disappears in time.
- Sometimes a fever occurs a few hours after the injection.
- Serious reactions are extremely rare.

Adults Beware if Not Immunised

Poliomyelitis is not just a childhood illness, it can affect anyone. Children in the UK for example, have been immunised against poliomyelitis since 1958. Those who were born before 1958 may not have been immunised. All adults who are not immunised against poliomyelitis should start by having the primary course of three poliomyelitis vaccines at monthly intervals. Then have the refresher doses as described above.

Travellers

Due to immunisation, poliomyelitis is almost eradicated from most parts of the world. However, it is still a problem in some regions, particularly Nigeria, Pakistan and other parts of Africa and Asia. GPs/physicians can advise on travel destinations for particular poliomyelitis risk areas should persons be travelling to such an area:

- Most persons will already be fully immunised from their routine childhood immunisations and do not need a refresher.

- If you have not had a refresher within the last 10 years, you may be advised to have a refresher dose of vaccine if you travel to certain countries. This is particularly important for health workers who intend to work in risk areas.

- Adults - see poliomyelitis vaccination notes above. If you are not immunised, you should be immunised before you travel.

Endemic Poliomyelitis Cases

Based on an estimated 350,000 cases, the endemic poliomyelitis cases have fallen since 1988 by more than 99% in more than 125 countries. In 2013, only parts of three countries in the world have not been declared poliomyelitis-free, the smallest geographic area in history. The number of cases of wild poliomyelitis virus type 3 have fallen to the lowest ever measured figures in history.

Other Parts of the Combined Vaccination

Tetanus

Tetanus is a serious bacterial infection that affects the nervous system, leading to painful muscle contractions, particularly of the jaw and neck muscles, also referred to as *lockjaw*.

Tetanus can interfere with the ability to breathe and can result in death. Cases of tetanus are rare in the developed world thanks to the tetanus vaccine but the incidence is much higher in developing countries. Approximately one million cases occur worldwide every year.

Tetanus is contracted through animal bites, burns, 'puncture wounds' – splinters, body piercings, tattoos, injected drugs – and even gunshot wounds have all been associated with tetanus infections.

Tetanus is the only vaccine-preventable disease that is infectious but is not contagious, meaning that it cannot be contracted from someone who has the disease once you have been vaccinated. The bacterium that causes tetanus (*Clostridium tetani*) is found in soil, dust and animal faeces, especially horse manure. The disease is caused by the bacteria entering a flesh wound, where it can start to produce a nerve toxin that affects nerves controlling your muscles.

Diphtheria

Diphtheria is an infectious disease affecting the nose, throat and sometimes the skin. It is caused by a bacterium that is spread through coughing and sneezing.

People usually become ill two to three days after becoming infected. Symptoms range from a moderately sore throat to toxic life-threatening diphtheria of the larynx or of the lower and upper respiratory tracts.

Diphtheria is often complicated, causing damage to heart muscles, kidneys or peripheral nerves from the toxin produced by the bacteria. It is fatal in up to 10% of cases.

Whooping Cough

Whooping cough is a highly contagious bacterial infection of the lungs and airways.

The medical term for whooping cough is Pertussis. The condition usually begins with a persistent dry and irritating cough, which progresses to intense bouts of coughing. These are followed by a distinctive *'whooping'* noise, which is how the condition gets its name.

Whooping cough is caused by a bacterium called *Bordetella pertussis*, which can be passed from person to person through droplets in the air from coughing and sneezing. Other symptoms include a runny nose, raised temperature and vomiting after coughing. The coughing can last for about three months (another name for whooping cough is the *hundred day cough*).

If whooping cough is diagnosed during the first three weeks (21 days) of infection, a course of antibiotics may be prescribed. This is to prevent the infection being passed on to others.

Babies under the age of six months are likely to be admitted to hospital as they are at most risk of having severe complications, such as serious breathing difficulties. They will be treated in isolation to prevent the infection spreading and will be given antibiotics into a vein through a drip (intravenously).

Poliomyelitis – History

Poliomyelitis infections extend into prehistory. Over millennia, polio-myelitis survived quietly as an endemic pathogenic until the 1880s when major epidemics began to occur in Europe.

The virus is spread in human waste. It is believed that the general introduction of hygiene in the late 19th century is one of the causes.

⟹ Less contact (*no immunization*), ⟹ more prone to catching the virus.

Poliomyelitis is caused by an intestinal virus infection that can lead to paralysis or death. The infection spread gradually over the world reaching the USA. In the first half of the 20th century, Europe was hit by severe epidemics.

By 1910, poliomyelitis epidemics became frequent events throughout the world and reached a peak in the 1940s and 1950s, when polio-myelitis killed or paralyzed over half a million people each year. Historical relics show that poliomyelitis had many victims even up to and over 5000 years ago.

Gamma globulin of the blood plasma of poliomyelitis survivors tested between 1951 and 1952 that contained poliomyelitis virus antibodies, gave promise of halting the poliomyelitis virus infection, but the Salk vaccine consisting of dead poliomyelitis virus carried out in mass vaccinations in the USA, Great Britain and Scandinavia from 1955/56 onwards, proved more successful. Albert Sabin developed an oral poliomyelitis vaccine (OPV) using live but weakened (*attenuated*) viruses. This was tested on humans from 1957 and licensed in 1962.

Germany:

Due to the persistence of the regional governments of Bavaria and North Rhine Westphalia mass vaccinations were first carried out in Germany in 1962. Until then, the German government had been in indecision with the health insurance companies over many years as to who was to pay for the vaccinations. During this time, from 1956 to the start of the German mass vaccinations in 1962, thousands of German children and adults were unfortunately infected by the virus. The first vaccinations against the extremely dangerous Type I poliomyelitis virus were then carried out and in the following years against type II and III. Since 1965 the trivalent vaccine against all 3 Serum types is in use.

Post-poliomyelitis Syndrome – PPS

Origin and Cause of Illness

PPS is a *neuro-degenerative illness*. Numerous theories have been proposed to explain PPS. The most widely accepted theory (based on medical studies) of the mechanism behind the disorder is *neural fatigue*, which seems to lay in the destruction of the remaining motor nerve cells due to overstressing (overload) over many years.

The reason being for this lies in the continuous additional stress on the remnant nerve cell bodies (giant motor nerve cell units formed after the acute illness), triggered by the physical and metabolic stress (high accumulation of excitatory nerve transmitters) to support and re-model the additional fibres that have been supporting more muscle fibres.

This had already been suggested by Wiechers and Hubbell from the state university of Ohio in Columbus in the early 1980s. According to their research, they found out that during an advanced number of years after the convalescence period, the motor nerve cells of polio-myelitis survivors increasingly lost their functional abilities.

Other causes that have been proposed by medical experts, whereby the evidence supporting these theories is extremely limited:

- a persistent infection of some kind,
- environmental chemicals, etc.

During the phase of functional stability, a continuous dysfunction of alpha motor nerve cells can be determined. According to current knowledge – once a certain threshold (destruction of more than ap-prox. 50% of the alpha motor nerve cells) is exceeded then this re-sults in a decompensation of the de- and re-innervation process that was started after the acute phase of poliomyelitis.

The de-compensation is pre-programmed, because under normal everyday conditions, the damaged nerve structures are already working on, or over their upper load limit and it is only a question of time, depending on the initial damage and the height of the overload before de-compensation takes place.

PPS Classification

Currently, PPS is classified as an independent disease (secondary illness). It possesses its own index G14 within the world wide ICD-10 definition (*International Classification of Disease*). In this respect it is distinguished – defined by the WHO (**W**orld **H**ealth **O**rganisation) in relation to all other after effects of poliomyelitis (ICD-10 **B91**).

When does the Post-poliomyelitis Syndrome Occur?

PPS manifests itself usually 15-40 years after an endured poliomyelitis in an acute or creeping form. It often begins with new weaknesses in muscles, where muscle contraction occurs repeatedly e.g. when walking, climbing the stairs and/or dressing. The weaknesses can also apply to muscles that were apparently not affected by the acute poliomyelitis. Breathing problems often arise for the first time in conjunction with an anaesthetic.

In most cases patients are treated with pain killers or other   medication, as most doctors or patients don't attribute the current status to the original poliomyelitis illness. Physical therapy (muscle building training), is very often prescribed, which is more harmful than helpful for the patient by speeding up the degeneration process.

It is presumed, that PPS is caused after the initial acute poliomyelitis by the **systematic overburden (overload)** over many decades of the few remaining motor nerve cells that perish irreversibly, one after the other.

As PPS cannot be healed, it is therefore most important to **accept the status** by taking it into consideration and changing and fitting the new situation into an entirely new way of life.

The Degeneration Path – (PPS)

More than approx. 95% of all spinal cord motor nerve cells and many brain cells can be stricken by the poliomyelitis infection. Some of them recover later on and others die.

The human organism can compensate partly for the loss of some motor nerve cells, but to what extent a paralysis remains cannot be foreseen. This is due to an inexplicable stimulation factor – numerous motor nerve cells that survive are able to make contact with abandoned muscle cells in their near vicinity, whereas the abandoned muscle cells would otherwise degenerate and die.

It is as though the body wants to keep as many of the muscle fibres that were uncoupled from the central control alive and functional. In the end, such a motor nerve cell that originally had innervations with perhaps 100-2000 individual muscle fibres then makes contact with 3000, 5000 or even 10,000 or more (building of giant motor nerve cell units).

This happens during the recovery phase and thereafter. The few surviving motor units take over the work of many of the abandoned motor nerve cells to form the giant motor nerve cell units.

However, this means that the remaining motor nerve cells work on a continuous power limit or even above (as if they were participating in a lifelong marathon race).

Our well-known graphic illustration below shows how the degeneration continues with PPS:

Degeneration ⇨ PPS

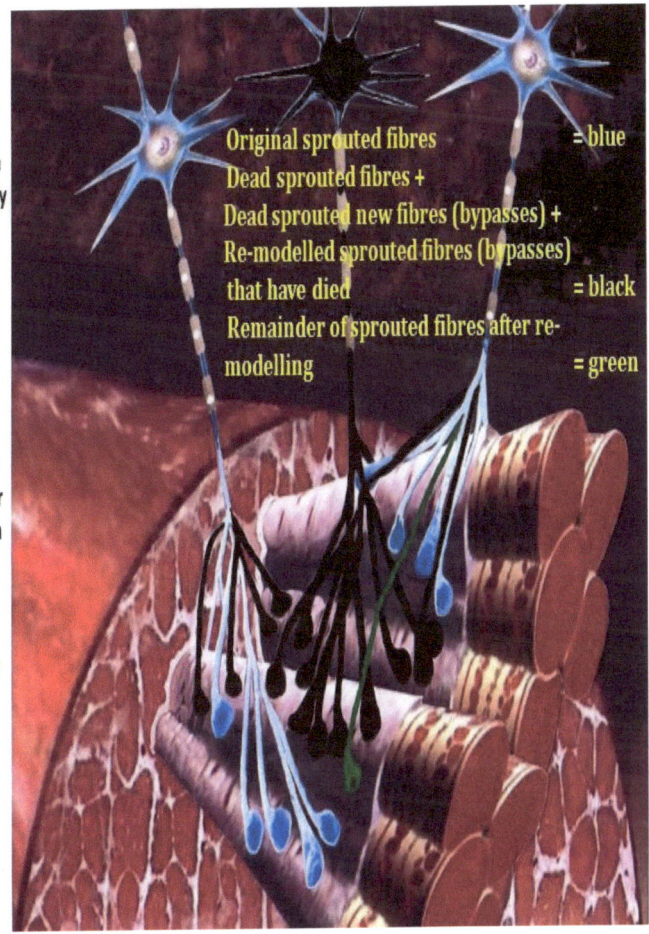

After many years (approx. 15 to 40) of a certain stability of body functions, the giant motor units start to degenerate. The consequences are a renewed muscle weakness.

Degeneration means that losses are greater than the regeneration can cope with.

Only the blue and green sprouted fibres have survived.

Original sprouted fibres = blue
Dead sprouted fibres +
Dead sprouted new fibres (bypasses) +
Re-modelled sprouted fibres (bypasses)
that have died = black
Remainder of sprouted fibres after re-modelling = green

PPS Symptoms

Health problems of the poliomyelitis survivors concerned in %

Tiredness	85
Muscular pains	80
Joint pains	80

General weakness

In previous stricken muscles	80
In muscles not previously stricken	60
Cold intolerance	45
Atrophies	35

Activity problems in daily life

Walking	75
Stair climbing	70
Dressing	40

Other symptoms

There are many other symptoms, such as urinary or bowel problems that may not be related to PPS. When other possible causes are ruled out, PPS is sometimes thought to be the case.

PPS Diagnosis

The diagnosis of the Post-poliomyelitis Syndrome (PPS), is based essentially on a detailed anamnesis, a thorough medical examination, including a neurological and orthopaedic status. There are no existing laboratory tests that give diagnostic proof.

The diagnosis of PPS is always an exclusion process that does not as such, give proof. Contrary endeavours in daily practice only prove the lack of specific knowledge of physicians.

Differential diagnostic examinations and laboratory procedures can be of diagnostic help. Computed tomography (CT), magnetic resonance imaging (MRI), electro-myogramm (EMG), ultra-sound, histological and laboratory tests could be useful in the determination process.

Muscular stress can often be recognised by an increase of the CK-MM* activity in serum (CK-MM = the muscle enzyme creatine kinase).

* The enzyme CK (creatine kinase), found primarily in the muscles, is important for the energy supply of the cells. One determines the CK in the blood for indications of skeletal muscle damage and myocardial damage (e.g. heart attack). In healthy subjects, the CK activity in the blood originates almost exclusively from skeletal muscle. CK may rise significantly on muscle damage. Increases of CK being released from other tissues rarely occurs.

The following indications give helpful references for a PPS diagnosis. However, they are not proof :

1.   A history of poliomyelitis is indicated in the anamnesis.

2.   After the acute illness, an improvement occurred.

3.   A stable phase of at least 10 years followed.

4.   Acute or new ailments start to creep up, or general deterioration, i.e.:

       -    On minimum activity, abnormal fatigue and exhaustion occurs.
       -    New muscular weaknesses and muscular atrophy.
       -    Progressive muscle, joint and nerve pains.
       -    Unusual temperature intolerance especially cold intolerance.
       -    Problems swallowing and sleep related disorders (nocturnal sleep apnoea).
       -    Problems after an anaesthetic, especially if the poliomyelitis illness was not considered when the type of anaesthetic and dose was applied.

5.   The neurological examination is compatible to a preceded poliomyelitis.

6.   All other diagnostics as an explanation for the new complaints can be sufficiently excluded.

Therapies – Post-poliomyelitis Syndrome

Fundamental Principles of Physiotherapy - PPS

Generally, an unbelievable, sometimes even frightening unawareness prevails in the application of an optimal physiotherapy for patients in a poliomyelitis late stadium, or with the PPS. This is often detrimental and occasionally even dangerous for the well-being and general health of the patients. The widely spread, ancient treatment slogan, in application many decades ago for patients suffering from an acute illness of poliomyelitis (infantile paralysis) was: maximum muscle training for the re-establishment of mobility according to the motto: *„practice, practice, practice and practice again"*, and is:

Unfortunately still being applied.

Due to the massive vaccination campaigns in the 1950's and 60's, poliomyelitis was practically driven out from medical everyday life in our modern world. The knowledge regarding this infection with its dire consequences and therapy went into oblivion and it was hardly ever taught. However, in the last couple of decades many new findings regarding the poliomyelitis late stages and the so-called Post-poliomyelitis Syndrome have been made. These important realizations:

"what one should do" and *"what one should rather not do",*

are not only in the physiotherapy departments of our medical establishments (i.e. small and general hospitals, clinics, universities, including rehabilitation establishments and physiotherapy schools), not really understood, but to an even larger extent, generally unknown.

The basis of an optimal physiotherapy for such patients defined in this booklet is in accordance with the current standards of science, technology and long-term experience – *state of the art.* A considerable amount of the neuro-physiological therapy conditions mentioned herein are not generally in practise by some therapists in their daily work and will therefore be regarded with more emphasis and described in greater detail.

Physiological Functioning After the Illness

☺ *(First of all, let's have a recap to freshen-up what we've learnt!)* ☺

The paralytical form of infantile paralysis results in *flaccid* paralyses, meaning: destruction of motor nerve cells in the front horn of the spinal cord, the so-called alpha motor nerve cells and their associated muscle fibres.

During the recovery phase (after the acute infection phase), new nerve cell sprouts, from remaining still intact motor nerve cell strings, sprout-out and innervate the muscle fibres that were previously innervated by the destroyed nerve cell sprouts. This means that they take over the tasks of the destroyed motor nerve cells and their corresponding nerve strings whose end sprouts were previously innervating those muscle fibres.

To explain that more simply: new nerve string sprouts from motor nerve cells already innervating neighbouring muscle fibres near the ones destroyed are formed and innervate as far as possible, the abandoned muscle fibres (replacement to a certain extent).

A distinct, but usually incomplete, muscular recovery phase occurs. This natural repairing procedure functions quite effectively. If a cell had to supply (innervate) just a few muscle cells before the infection, it now has to supply some hundreds or even thousands more. This becomes a so-called *giant motor unit* and thus the area of responsibility and metabolism of the particular nerve cell in this process increases in size immensely.

Clinically, a clear improvement of muscle power occurs and in the follow-up phase, many poliomyelitis patients are able to move or perhaps even run better than before.

Even after and due to the acute illness, further problems may occur. Since children still in the growth phase are generally affected by the illness, a different growth of the extremities due to the different paralysis-related weight-loading and the different use of the extremities results. For example, an arm badly affected can become frail and shorter than the other arm that may not have been affected by the infection or perhaps only slightly. In the spinal cord area, deformations and scoliosis caused by weaknesses in the trunk musculature may occur. Likewise, contractures due to the weight-load differences may occur.

Typically, after a long period of functional and neurological stability of about 15 – 40 years (sometimes less), approximately 70% of the patients who suffered poliomyelitis in their childhood start to have problems in the form of:

-       Renewed weaknesses (loss of strength and endurance).
-       Increased **exhaustion** (not connected to over-straining).
-       Endurance decrease and functional loss, including pain increase, particularly in the muscles and joints.
-       Muscle atrophy.
-       Breathing difficulties.
-       Swallowing and speech difficulties.
-       Increased cold intolerance.

The patients have increased difficulties in mastering the daily requirements of life (work pressure/excessive demands). The so-called Post-poliomyelitis Syndrome (PPS), medically defined as an independent secondary illness, sets in. PPS has its own index G14 within the world-wide ICD-10 definition (International Classification of Disease). The causes of the PPS have not yet been finally clarified. The most probable cause considered is an overloading and consequently the destruction of remaining motor nerve cells caused through metabolic stress. During the functional stability phase, a continued dysfunction of the alpha-motor nerve cells can be determined. According to the current medical doctrine, if a certain threshold (destruction of more than 50-60% of the motor nerve cells) is exceeded, the Post-poliomyelitis Syndrome occurs due to the decompensation of the de- and re-innervation process that has been happening since the acute poliomyelitis phase.

Neurological Clinical Findings

On ascertaining the initial status before the start of   therapeutic physical treatment, the following findings should be taken into consideration:

1. A variable picture of flaccid paralyses is apparent throughout, whereby the paralysis picture is not symmetrical but varied and usually proximately accentuated. With PPS, muscles not previously affected by the earlier poliomyelitis can also be clinically affected. It is in discussion that these could be groups of muscles that were sub-clinical, thus not visibly affected by the poliomyelitis.

2. Skeleton deformities (extremities and/or spinal cord) resulting in long term postural damage are apparent. Therefore the passive holding and inter-locking mechanisms are often over-loaded, resulting in increasingly unstable joints, increased wear and pain, accompanied by a correspondingly defective posture. Due to the compensation mechanisms then practised, further structures, at that point apparently healthy, become additionally over-loaded and damaged.

3. Vague muscular pains, difficult to characterize – above all, and **especially** at night.

4. Joint contractures.

5. Breathing problems with respiratory insufficiency (spontaneous breathlessness and after exertion), also sleep apnoea syndrome.
    The breathing insufficiency is caused both by the PPS conditioned disturbances of the breathing centre in the brain stem and/or the damage of the alpha-motor nerve cells in the spinal cord responsible for the respiratory muscles (that resulted in a weakening) and can be aggravated too by mechanical hindrance caused by scoliosis.
    It usually crops up for the first time after infections of the respiratory system or longer lasting anaesthesia.

6. An abnormal temperature intolerance, mostly cold intolerance

7. Often distinctive lymphatic edema on both legs due to the inactivity of the leg musculature (wheelchair user), also in some cases without explainable reason (thus idiopathic).

8.   Occasional swallowing disturbances with increased aspiration risk, dysphagia, dysarthria and hoarseness.

9.   Occasionally nerve lesions (e.g. carpal tunnel syndrome) - usually due to secondary damage especially caused by the use of help-aids in particular.

10. Occasional osteoporosis.

Selection of a Suitable Therapy

Due to the pathophysiological precondition and the initial nerve-muscular status of the patient in the selection of an optimal individual therapy, the following criteria should always be considered **before** the start of a therapy:

1. Poliomyelitis and the Post-poliomyelitis Syndrome *are neurological illnesses* and therefore *require a neurologically oriented therapy*. Primary designated orthopaedic training therapies generally prescribed are **not helpful** and therefore **not indicated.**

2. Muscle building therapies are generally seen as **obsolete**, as they cause a further overloading of the alpha motor nerve cells. This unnecessary additional overload can cause a speeded-up exodus of the nerve cell(s).

3. Muscle preserving therapies however are indicated.

4. The therapy must be carried out considerately. Should a muscular cramp or strain arise as a result, then the therapy was too intensive. As a consequence the therapy must be reduced.

5. The treatment plan arranged for each patient must be of a strict individual nature, because the paralytic patterns vary from patient to patient, also the difference in the disease process, including the diversity and difference in living and working conditions over the last decades, the use of aids (or-theses, manually driven wheelchairs, electric wheelchairs etc.). Therefore, fixed or schematized treatment programs, as well as treatment in groups **are not generally indicated**, mostly ineffective, in fact pointless and therefore useless and a waste of valuable resources.

6. The patient must be guided and controlled via direct contact with the therapist during the course of all therapies. This means e.g. that in aqua movement therapies, the therapist must also be present with the patient in the water. An optical control from the side of the baths, is unfortunately still too often in practice and therapeutic nonsense.

Optimal Physical Therapeutical Treatment Concept

In order to achieve the optimal physical therapeutic treatment goal for this particular clientele, a coordinated concept should at least include the following areas:

○ Preservation of muscle functions and coordination.

○ Relaxation and improvement of the muscle metabolism.

○ Contracture and scoliosis prophylaxis.

○ Vegetative stimulation.

○ Functional training.

○ Help aids – supply and training.

○ Respiration therapy.

The following principles for physical therapy with PPS patients should be followed. *[modified according to Gusowski (2012)]:*

○ The holistic assessment of the patient and his problems as opposed to an emphasis on the treatment of individual body structures should be held foremost.

○ Participation oriented goal.

○ Relief therapy as opposed to endurance training.

○ Re-coordination of the muscles is more important than body-building.

○ Economization of movement.

○ Reactive- and reflex therapeutic approach, rather than more intense related resistance exercises.

○ Contracture and prevention of spinal curvature (scoliosis prophylaxis).

○ Relaxation and improvement of muscle metabolism.

○ Help-aids testing, supply and training.

○ Making sure of the usage of help-aids instead of exhaustion (it doesn't make sense when the patient is completely exhausted on appearance for therapy).

Suitable Therapies

A prerequisite on the selection of the therapy forms with this particular clientele, is that a careful *muscle-preserving* treatment is to be applied and *not a muscle building* treatment. An important ruling requirement here:

"Coordination before strength!"

The following are therapy types that have worked particularly well over many years:

- ° Relaxation therapy: improvement of the muscle metabolism.
- ° Positioning: comfortable starting/sitting position, in a wheelchair, seating ergonomics.
- ° Sling table treatment.
- ° Movement bath (34 ° C water temperature).
- ° Massages: these however, **should not** lead to the lowering of the muscular tension in such a way that the patient has problems, therefore being forced to increase his compensation mechanisms.
- ° Relaxation therapies: e.g. Jacobson, in addition, Yoga etc.
- ° Interference current: particularly on pain indication.
- ° Heat treatment.
- ° Specific application of help-aids.
- ° Muscle preservation and co-ordination.
- ° Stimulation techniques.
- ° Isometric exercises.
- ° Working in facilitation systems.

Treatment Plan

☺ *Remember:* ☺

The treatment plan arranged for each patient must be of a strict individual nature, because the paralytic patterns vary from patient to patient, also the difference in the infection process, including the diversity and difference in living and working conditions over the last decades, the use of aids (orthesis, manually driven wheelchairs, electrical wheelchairs etc.). Therefore, fixed or schematized treatment programs, as well as treatment in groups are not generally indicated, mostly ineffective, in fact pointless and therefore useless and a waste of valuable resources.

Experience has shown that a combination of many well-known and accepted treatment methods (parts or excerpts thereof) on an individual basis is extremely important. Hereby, the best results for patient relief and maintaining the current PPS status without further physically damaging (decimating) the remaining re-innervated nerve string sprouts must be the main aim and can be achieved.

Some Treatment Methods:

Bobath
Brunkow
PNF
Vojta
Feldenkrais, etc.

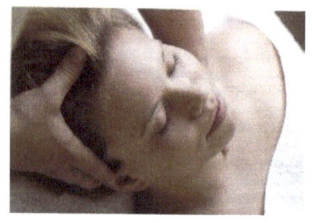 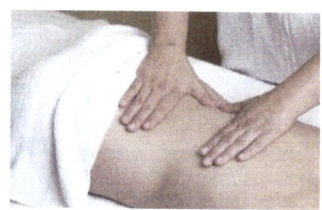

Movement baths
(34° C Water temperature)

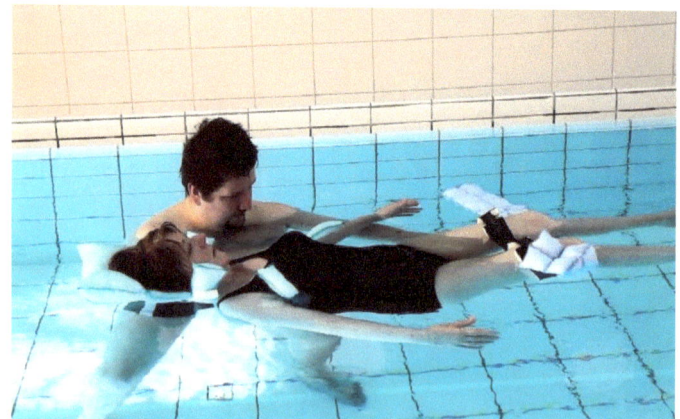

Anaesthesia/Operation

The Patient

The patient should know that knowledge of PPS amongst physicians is often very limited: there is little literature on PPS. Internet searches are rarely carried out and communication with self-help groups doesn't take place very often. Therefore, PPS demands teamwork between anaesthetists, surgeons, physiotherapists, nurses and patients.

The patient should offer the anaesthetist information (literature, booklets, internet link addresses) and communicate on an eye-to-eye level. The patient should speak openly about issues, fears and problems and possibly involve the partner or self-help group. The aspiration to work together in a trustworthy way with the anaesthetist is important.

Only this cooperation between patient and anaesthetist with mutual acceptance on the same level and the efforts made for an optimal exchange of information before surgery, can contribute to an optimal approach.

What should the Physician/Anaesthetist Know?

The clinical picture of the Post-poliomyelitis Syndrome is unfamiliar to many physicians/anaesthetists. A customized surgical OP plan according to the patient's disease related disabilities, as well as for follow-up treatment after the OP, should be made. An intensive and careful preparation even in apparently healthy, respectively muscular compensated PPS patients, is very important for safety reasons during the operating phase.

What does the Anaesthetist Need to Know ?

The anaesthetist should have basic knowledge about poliomyelitis, i.e. that this particular illness causes the destruction of alpha-motor front horn cells through virus infestation – that the cervical and lumbar spinal cord regions are particularly affected – that approximately two thirds of the illness are of spinal form and a third of bulbar and bulbospinal form. A combination of both forms is also possible.

Some PPS patients have a general consistent anxiety before surgery and the associated anaesthesia, especially those patients who have previously experienced the latter.

In comparison to other patients, PPS patients require a longer recovery time and a longer convalescence.

There are other features that the doctor/anaesthetist needs to know about PPS patients.

What the Physician/Anaesthetist Should Know About the PPS Patient:

- Which muscles were affected during the acute poliomyelitis infection and in what form?
- What was the state after the recovery/regeneration?
- After the poliomyelitis infection: was artificial respiration applied to the patient, or did the patient have a respiratory weakness, or was the patient in the iron lung?
- What restrictions exist currently?
- What other illnesses and limitations does the patient have?
- Which medicines/painkillers does the patient have to take and what medication intolerance does the patient have?

The Anaesthetist Should Know about the Main PPS Symptoms:

- Paralyses (also renewed) and weaknesses of the musculature.
- Breathing problems.
- Increased frequency of obstructive and central sleep apnoea.
- Weakness of the pharyngeal muscles with dysphagia.
- Cold intolerance.
- Medication intolerance.
- Pain in muscles and joints.
- Rapid tiredness.
- Chest deformity.

This means above all:

"Communication between patient and physician on the same level."

The patient informs the physician through literature or via self-help groups and makes his individual needs be heard (e.g. physical therapy, respiratory therapy, sensitivities, etc.). Discussions about the anaesthesia procedures are permitted and desired.

Physicists/Anaesthetist – Before the Operation:

How does the Anaesthetist Have to React ?

The risks of the anaesthesia and operation must be included in the operational planning. It is to be noted that PPS patients have lesser muscle mass and require lesser medication dosage but have an increased demand for blood and liquids and that quite often breathing problems are foremost. Medication sensitivity is extremely high, particularly with narcotics and anaesthetics.

Muscle relaxants should be avoided. In addition, the patient has an increased contact-, pressure-, pain- and temperature- sensitivity. Accordingly, the positioning of the patient is very important.

The anaesthetist should take into account that intubation problems can occur and that quite often cold intolerance is present and heating application is indicated.

An immediate physical therapy – passive movement exercises on a neuro-physiological basis should take place directly postoperative – early mobilization should be done gently (muscle-sparing -> passive).

The anaesthetist should also take into consideration that a PPS patient has perhaps more information about PPS and most probably over a longer period, so that the instructional part regarding the operation and dangers thereby should be approached on the same level as the patient.

The administration of antacids (e.g. 300 mg ranitidine PO) on the evening before and on the day of surgery prior to surgery – a preventive measure of postoperative nausea and vomiting (after surgery) is recommended.

Medication:

Many PPS patients have relapsing (frequent/permanent) pain and are familiar with painkillers.

Register the effectiveness of medication!
(Increased opioid sensitivity)

Blood Reserves:

Due to lesser muscle mass with PPS patients and significant paralyses, a reduced blood volume exists **(blood reserves)**.

Premedication

Drugs for premedication should have a soothing/anti-anxiety effect (sedative/anxiolytic), **no muscle relaxant**s (e.g. Promethazine, Opipramol or alpha-2 agonists).

In extremity surgery of the peripheral, nerve blockades or regional processes are of an advantage!

Surgery Day

Effective for all anaesthesia procedures: active heat measures, especially on an existing cold intolerance.

Regional Anaesthesia

A deterioration of the neurological situation after regional anaesthesia is possible. The decision for or against this procedure is made by the anaesthesiologist who weighs the potential pros and cons!

For regional anaesthesia: if necessary, reduce the applied amount of the local anaesthetic – peripheral and central regional anaesthesia using catheter techniques (in addition to a general anaesthesia). This facilitates postoperative opioid-free pain therapy.

General Anaesthesia

When general anaesthesia is considered: preferably no muscle relaxants – usage of a laryngeal mask – as few opioids as possible – use generally well controlled, short-effective substances.

Here is an Example that Fulfils the Anaesthesia Criteria:

Initiation:

Anaesthesia induction Propofol 1-2 mg/kg body weight
Fentanyl 2 micrograms/kg body weight
Muscle relaxation Mivacurium 0.2 mg/kg body weight

Anaesthesia:

Remifentanil 0.05-0.2 micrograms/kg body weight/min
Desflurane or Sevoflurane 0.4-0.8 MAC
Post relaxation only neuromuscular monitoring
Multimodal PONV prophylaxis (4 mg Dexamethasone, 4 mg Ondansetron, 0.5 mg Haloperidol)
supplementation, if need be, with alpha-2 agonists
Start pain therapy!
(1.5 g Novalminsulfon and Piritramid at reduced doses)

Waking-up Phase:

Aspirate mouth/throat, check residual relaxation and antagonize if necessary.

On termination of the anaesthesia, anaesthetics and analgesics should be stopped early. Regional anaesthesia should be continued without local anaesthetics.

Muscle power measurement by means of relax-meter: waking-up phase with respiration support.

Postoperative Phase

- Continuous monitoring of vital signs in the recovery room (extended monitoring).
- Breathing exercises, invitation to cough, if necessary (patient to bring personal apparatus) CPAP. Ventilatory support and physiotherapy should be done on a neuro-physical basis and early mobilization take place on the day of operation.
- Head of bed elevation 30 ° (for aspiration prophylaxis).
- Thermal action (warmth).
- Pain: opioids carefully titrated (choice and dosage), combined with non-opioids, preferably regional anaesthesia procedures with patient controlled analgesia (PCA) (pain absence control).
- Provide indication for monitoring on intermediate care or intensive care unit generously.

Important:

As a rule, the recovery phase of poliomyelitis survivors takes much longer.

Post-poliomyelitis Syndrome - Every Step Counts

When are Humans Healthy?

When they are in motion! This is necessary for the soul that would purge into neurotic rigidity, if it didn't swing to the rhythm of a healthy life with sufficient social-emotional inspirations. Still more for the body that would suffer decay, if stuck in a prison of movement retard.

The WHO defined a minimum of 150 minutes of *moderate movement* per week as a protection means from chronic civilisation illnesses (above all, heart-circulation weakness, diabetes, chest- and colon-cancer). Only one third of earthly citizens fulfil this demand. The number of the physically active doing it for vocational reasons sinks constantly, modern technology replacing the effort more and more.

Approximately 30% of the world population does not abide by the movement limit defined by the WHO.

With poliomyelitis survivors it is somewhat different. They are significantly limited in their ability to move and exercise their limbs and should not be overloaded. It is nevertheless very important that poliomyelitis survivors try to keep in active movement according to their individual capabilities.

Factors that Limit the Risk

Having to deal with an illness again, thought to have been part of the past, can be discouraging, even overwhelming at times. Recovering from the initial illness required drive and determination, but now the late effects of poliomyelitis require rest and a conservation of energy. Moving from one frame of mind to another can be difficult.

Here are some suggestions that may help:

Limit activities that cause pain or fatigue

Moderation is the key. Overdoing it on a good day can lead to several subsequent bad days.

Be smart

Conserving energy through lifestyle modifications and assistive devices doesn't mean giving in to the illness. It just means a smarter way has been found to deal with it.

Stay warm

Cold increases muscle fatigue. Keep your home at a comfortable temperature and dress in layers, especially when you go out.

Avoid falls

Get rid of throw rugs and loose clutter on the floor, wear good shoes and avoid slippery or icy surfaces.

Maintain a healthy lifestyle

Eat a balanced diet, don't smoke or stop smoking and decrease caffeine intake to keep fit, breathe easier and sleep better.

Protect your lungs

If your breathing is impaired, watch for signs of a developing respiratory infection, which can make breathing problems worse and have it treated promptly. Also, avoid smoking areas (don't smoke yourself to death either) and stay current with your flu and pneumonia vaccines.

Factors that Increase the Risk

Factors that may increase your risk of developing the Post-poliomyelitis Syndrome include:

Severity of the initial poliomyelitis infection

The more severe the initial infection, the more likely you'll have signs and symptoms of the Post-poliomyelitis Syndrome.

Age at onset of the initial illness

The older you were when you were infected by poliomyelitis, the greater the risk of developing PPS. For example, if you acquired poliomyelitis as an adolescent or adult, rather than as a young child, your chances of developing the Post-poliomyelitis Syndrome increase.

Recovery

The greater your recovery after the acute poliomyelitis infection, the more likely it seems that the Post-poliomyelitis Syndrome will develop. This is seen to be because greater recovery places additional stress on motor nerve cells (giant motor units).

Physical activity

If you perform physical activity to the point of exhaustion or fatigue more than often, this may overload already stressed-out motor nerve cells and increase your risk of a Post-poliomyelitis Syndrome.

Help Aids

Everyday life assistance serves the purpose of reaching and preserving the greatest possible independency and furthering of life quality!

"Mobility is an important part of our lives, regardless of age."

Whether you need domestic help aids or for general mobility: get more information! Inform yourself, for example, at a self-help group or health agency, or make internet enquiries before you purchase or apply for help aid(s).

Wheelchairs

Why and when do I need a wheelchair and how do I get one?

It mostly starts with the falls – for some time now you've been experiencing a weakness in the legs (support seems bad but only now and again. Prolonged standing is an ordeal and if you have to stand for more than a few minutes, then your mind goes into turmoil: *"any moment now my legs will collapse...,"* and in your mind, you see yourself falling. This may well happen.

You've been hesitant or reluctant about using help-aids. They don't seem to be an option to you. Why should they? You are really not that much in need, or so you try to induce yourself to think. Well, you're wrong because falls may end up with serious consequences!

You're out for a walk, walking slowly but surely. All of a sudden, in the leg that you have just moved forward, you have no more feeling of strength. You fall, hopefully without serious injury. It can happen anywhere, in the garden, in the bathroom, or in a place where dangerous things may be around you or on the ground. This could mean a serious injury for you, with serious consequences!

Although you have the feeling that there is still some strength left in the leg or legs. The truth is that the degeneration started many years ago and has progressed continuously. Together with this increase in acute instability you also experience an increase in muscle pain and cramping that temporarily or permanently deprives you of your sleep at night. The cramps also occur during the day, but you're used to them and have become capable of coping with the situation.

For many years now you've been experiencing pain in joints and tendons (part of the process of degeneration) and have great difficulty or even cessation of strength, a sort of paralytic feeling when walking. All in all you should ask yourself seriously if you perhaps are in need of a wheelchair or help-aid of some kind?

The wheelchair stigma

There is such a thing as a wheelchair stigma that might discourage you from using one. You don't want to just give up and get used to life in a wheelchair - what will people think of you? Once in a wheelchair, always in a wheelchair! That's nonsense! You only have to get used to the situation and it definitely does not necessarily mean that you then have to stay permanently in a wheelchair!

Many people seem *irritated* when they see a poliomyelitis survivor or MS   patient sitting regularly in a wheelchair and then seeing them suddenly walking about again and then a few days later back in the wheelchair again... and so on.

Some poliomyelitis survivors have difficulties coping with this fact – one day to be in a wheelchair and another day walking about with crutches or even to be walking about on foot without help-aids. Perhaps this is because they attach too much importance to the opinions of others. This too is nonsense! Use the wheelchair when necessary and on all occasions take your crutches with you.

If you are able to and if necessary, use your crutches for short distances and in your home or around it. If your arms are not yet affected, use a rollator/walker.

If you have an electrically powered wheelchair, then you may need a ramp(s) or a lift to load the wheelchair into your car. You should also have a manually operated wheelchair for short distances. If you are unable to use your arms then you'll need someone to push you.

It is advisable for poliomyelitis survivors who require a wheelchair, but do not yet have one, to seek advice from a nearby poliomyelitis help group or advisory authority, if possible. There are many pitfalls or rather important factors that must be considered. For example, if your arms are too weak, you will need an electric-powered wheelchair. If you live in an area where the slopes are extreme, you will need a particularly powerful electric wheelchair to get you up the gradients. Otherwise it may happen that you'll be given a wheelchair that is of no use to you.

When you apply for a wheelchair, ask for wheelchair training.

Some wheelchair examples

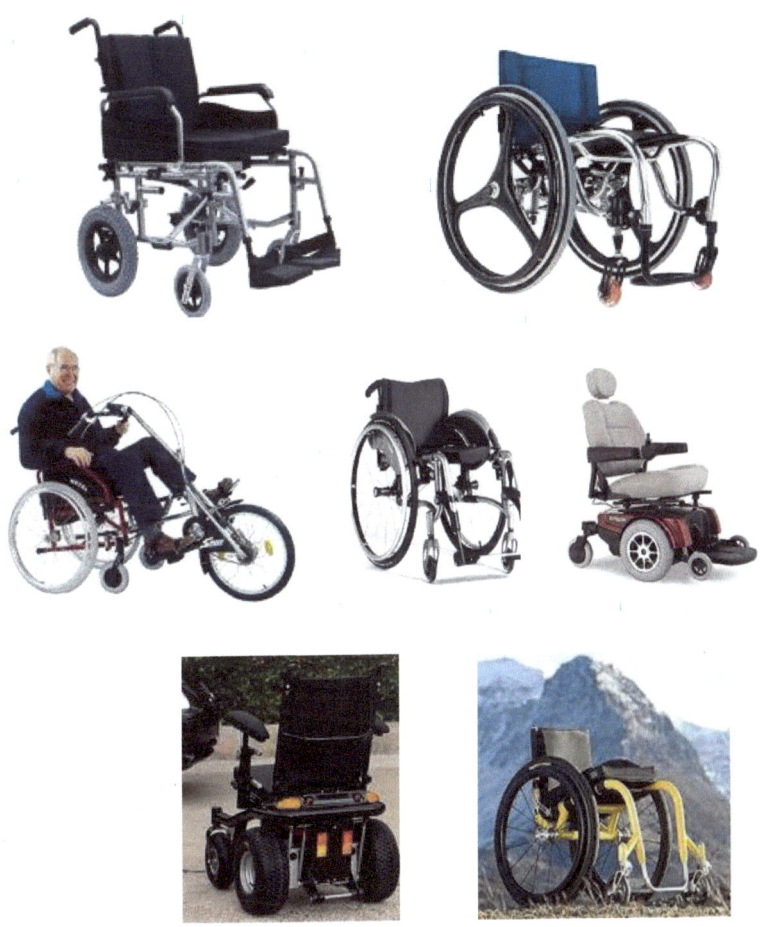

Orthoses

Orthotics (Greek: *ortho, to straighten* or *align*) is a speciality within the medical field concerned with the design, manufacture and application of orthoses. An *orthosis* (plural: *orthoses*) means: *an externally applied device used to modify the structural and functional characteristics of the neuromuscular and skeletal system.*

Orthoses can be used to:

- Restrict the control, or physical movement of a limb, and or joint or body part to immobilize it/them for a particular reason.

- In order to restrict movement in a certain direction.

- To support general movement.

- In order to reduce or compensate the weight of physical bearing forces for a particular purpose.

- For rehabilitation after a fracture, after the removal of the plaster to give the affected limb further support.

- To change the shape (distortion) and/or correct the function of a particular skeleton part and to offer an easier movement possibility, or to relieve pain.

Foot-joint orthosis - is used when a person suffers from a flaccid ankle as a result of injury to the peroneal nerve.

Orthotic shells – have a comfortable deep heel cup with a little intrusive arch profile

Classification

Orthoses are described using acronyms that classify the particular joints they affect. Such as a <u>F</u>oot <u>L</u>ifter <u>O</u>rthosis ('FLO') that affects the foot and ankle, or a <u>T</u>horacic <u>l</u>umbar <u>s</u>acral <u>o</u>rthosis ('TLSO') that affects the thoracic, lumbar and sacral regions of the spine.

Examples

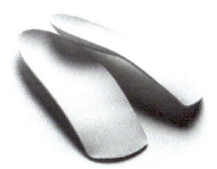 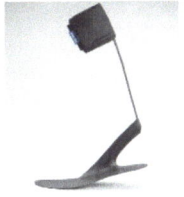 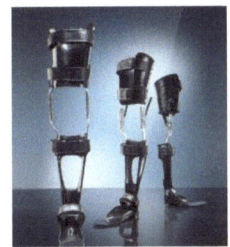

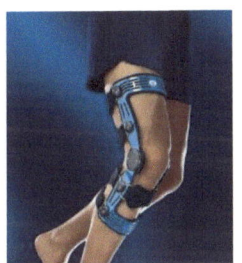 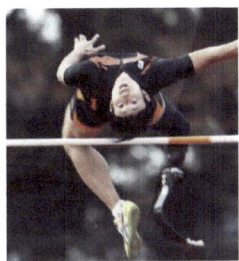 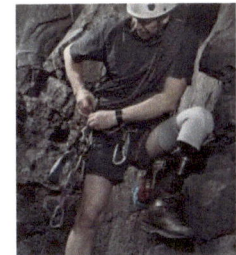

Walking Aids

Examples of walking aids:

Rollator, walker with frame, walking sticks, crutches, etc.:

Aluminium armpit crutches

Some armpit crutches feature patented clip-lock adjustable handles and push button foot pieces for fast, precise measuring and fitting. High-density rubber cushions and handgrips provide long wear and greater comfort and are made from light-weight aluminium. There are also a variety of other types of models, depending on the disability.

Shock absorbing crutches

Patented shock absorbing crutch systems within the crutches, help to reduce the strain on wrist, elbow and shoulder joints. Height adjustable between the handle and the ground and between handle and cuff, they can be tailored to fit a wide range of users. Aluminium and plastic constructions ensure that the crutches are lightweight and weigh approx. 600g.

Rollators:

There are two- and four-wheeled rollators, compact aluminium rollators etc. For two-wheeled rollators, rubber plugs are fixed to the rear rack feet. As a rule, four-wheeled rollators with a (collapsible) seating possibility and good brakes are used and recommended.

Walking sticks:

There are a variety of walking sticks, also lightweight collapsible-type models.

Some examples:

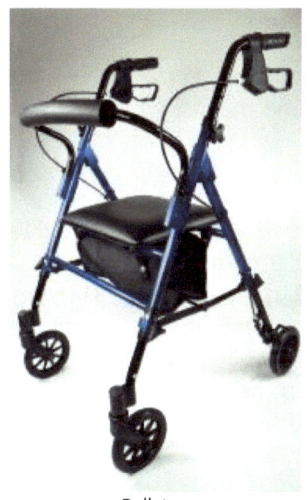

Rollator

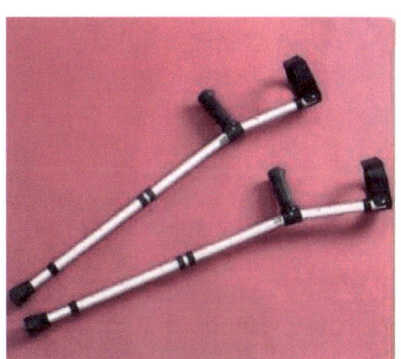

Shock absorbing crutches

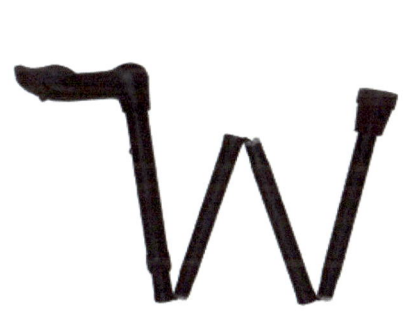

Foldable walking stick with arthritis grip

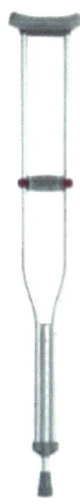

Armpit crutch

Bathroom Help-Aids

Some examples:

A few examples of handgrips, toilet seats, shower seats and bath lifters. There are many others on the market:

Toilet seat, toilet seat-safety frame

The toilet seat with safety frame is designed to provide maximum comfort for those who have problems going to the toilet. Such toilet seats have a vertical splash guard to avoid soiling. They also feature a large seating area with a recess channel in order to minimize the risk of sloshing.
In most cases, the seat-aid can be easily removed for hygienic cleansing or refitting. On some models, the seating aid is also suitable for bidet-use.

Bath lift

For people with reduced mobility, a bath lift is a wonderful way to ensure that the bathing experience is as safe and enjoyable as possible. The bath lift is normally easy to install and remove from the bath. Bath lifts have regular easy clean, hygienic surfaces. The covers are washable mostly to 60 degrees. Hand controls are waterproof, can float and mostly have a suction cup on the back, so that they can be placed within reach. There are strong, robust types available on the market that ensure maximum stability. They fit most bathtub sizes and shapes.

Other types of bath aids:

Padded shower benches, handrail grips, etc.

Some illustrated examples:

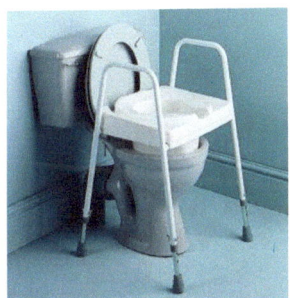

Toilet seat with safety frame

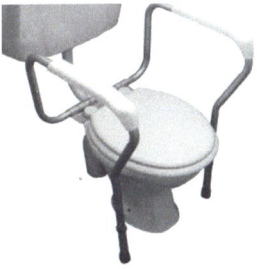

Toilet seat getting-up help-aid

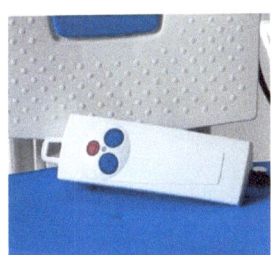

Bath lift – hand control

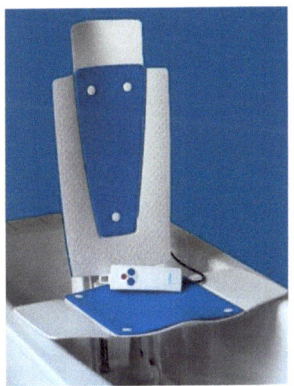

Bath lift

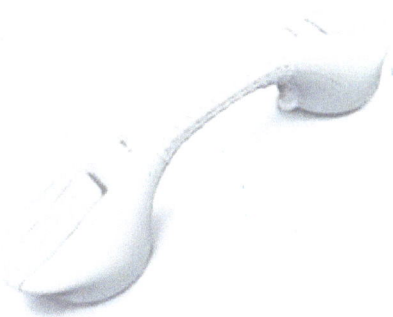

Handrail grip

Household Aids

Foldable gripping aid

Button-hook help

Zipper-gripper

Shoe remover

Compression stocking dressing help

Rotating gripper arm help, etc.

Some examples:

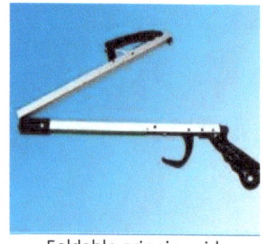
Foldable gripping aid

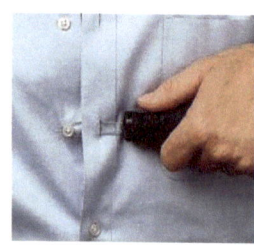
Button-hook help

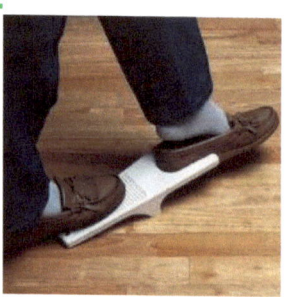
Shoe remover

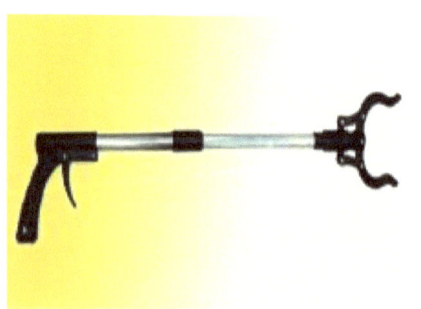
Rotating gripper-arm help aid

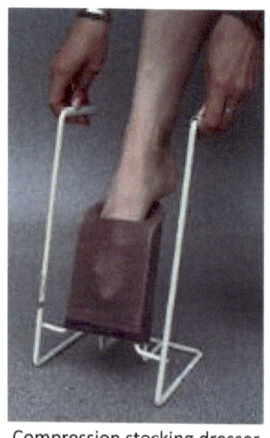
Compression stocking dresser

Kitchen Utensils

There are many types of adapted utensils, carving knives, gripping aids, scissors, forks and spatulas for the disabled or elderly, which are available on the market. These are designed with either special grips or blades for people with weak grip or limited range of motion.

Here are a few examples:

Carving knife: Has the benefit of a non-slip, ergonomically angled handle for increased comfort. Holding the black soft-feel non-slip handle, the knife can be used as normal. The angled handle keeps the wrist in a neutral position thus preventing strain whilst in use. A non-slip finish improves the grip even when a hand is wet or greasy.

One-hand container/box: The one-hand container/box is perfect for anyone with weak hands. The container/box is easy to open with no twisting or turning. To open, one has to simply press on the little spot on the rim of the lid with one finger or the flat of the hand. To reseal the container, one simply presses the middle of the lid.

Swivel peeler: The swivel peeler peels easily and requires minimal wrist movement. It has a regular stainless-steel blade and tapered, oversized hole for hanging-up. The handle ensures a secure hold, even when wet. It is safe for a household dishwasher.

Special grip help aids
Scissors
Forks
Can opener
Spatula
etc.

Some examples:

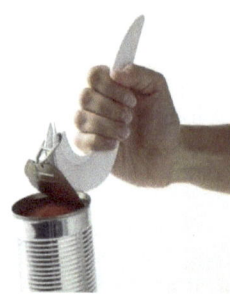

Can opener

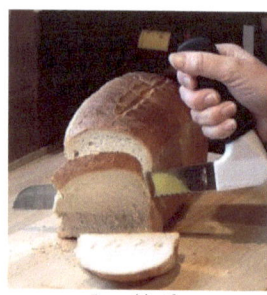

Bread knife

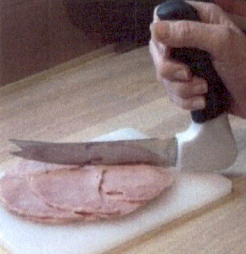

Carving knife – multi usage

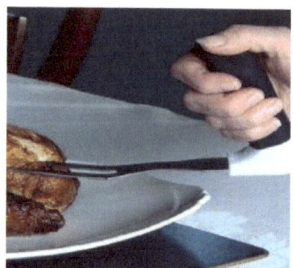

Carving fork

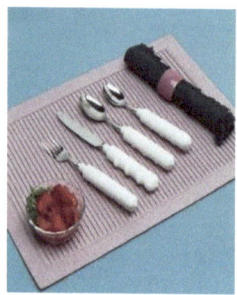

Cutlery with special handles

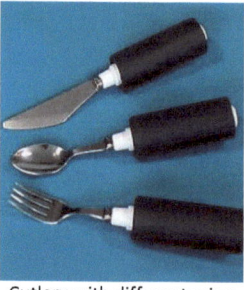

Cutlery with different grips

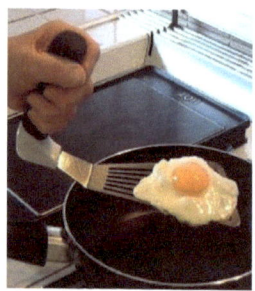

Spatula with special handle

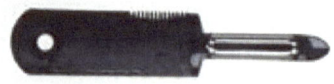

Swivel peeler

PPS Research

Western Europe was freed from poliomyelitis due to the massive vaccination programs (mainly in the form of the so-called *oral vaccine* of the 50s and 60s of the last century under the motto:

Oral vaccine is sweet, poliomyelitis is cruel.

Only sporadic isolated cases of poliomyelitis infections that had been introduced by tourists and migrants occurred occasionally.

Over the past four decades almost no more poliomyelitis infections could be observed by general practitioners and hospital clinics in Western Europe. Poliomyelitis disappeared almost completely from sight, from our consciousness and the focus of public attention – it had become a medical rarity. Unfortunately the knowledge and experience obtained concerning the illness also disappeared. Thus, there was no need for further knowledge of this ancient infectious disease in medical studies, medical specialist training, or generally to mediate the illness in medical programs and literature. Although we had amassed a very considerable amount of knowledge on poliomyelitis and in retrospect of current requirements, maintaining and updating this knowledge was unfortunately totally neglected. Poliomyelitis caught up with us profoundly over the last three decades in the form of poliomyelitis late effects, the so-called Post-poliomyelitis Syndrome (PPS).

Why the late effects after the initial poliomyelitis infection remained a relatively little explored medical field, is still not entirely clear. One reason may be that until now the realization is that a stone-dead nerve cell could never be revived by any researcher or doctor. The other reason may be due to the vaccinations – once the mass vaccinations eradicated the infectious disease it wasn't of importance for further research or monetary funding any more, thereby all those who were infected before the mass vaccinations took place just slipped into the category of being victims of a disease that from then on was avoidable through vaccination and nothing was really known, or the medical authorities were not unduly interested in any late effects that couldn't really be signified. Besides, most of those patients were treated with pain killers or other medication or even deemed to be malingerers, as most doctors or even the patients themselves didn't attribute their current status to the original poliomyelitis illness. The reason for research into the late effects only came into effect because some poliomyelitis patients were from the medical profession who then founded self-help groups, for which we poliomyelitis survivors are extremely grateful.

According to current knowledge, treatment using so-called *stem cells* cannot be carried out because the necessary infrastructure (in the central and peripheral nervous system, as well as in the muscles) is destroyed during the course of time after the acute infection, or reduced and mostly replaced by binding tissue. Newly sprouted nerve cells from stem cells are not able to find a way or reach the previously destroyed target organ muscle cells. Overall, there are currently very few academic institutions that are concerned with the elucidation of the disease-related-physiological processes of PPS. Few diseases have been so intensively researched as poliomyelitis. Because of the rapid and dramatic onset of symptoms, poliomyelitis was considered the classic example of an acute viral infectious disease. The majority of scientific energies and most resources were concentrated on early management and prevention, without any research area having dealt with the long-term effects or late effects. To date, the paralytic form of poliomyelitis found in medical textbooks is still being described as a static or stable neurological disease. That is, as we know today, in no way correct.

Although we have gained many new and very valuable insights into the aetiology and optimal treatment of PPS in recent decades, we obviously have not succeeded enough in establishing this knowledge in clinics, hospitals and GP practices. Knowledge for a qualified diagnosis and treatment of PPS patients by doctors and physio- therapists is usually zero. Most of them even claim that such a thing as PPS doesn't exist. Of course the ones who suffer the most, the PPS patients and their families, are very frustrated about the situation. Ignorance and lack of knowledge of the needs of PPS patients all too often lead to a denial of necessary treatments and the granting of aids. Thus, most PPS affected are forced to lead a life that becomes a busy and tiring fight for their rights. It still applies:

"Whoever was once infected by the polio-myelitis virus has a life-long fight ahead."

Of some help for poliomyelitis survivors are the more or less globally widespread poliomyelitis self-help organizations. These organizations, help according to the motto:

"Together we are strong"

They give enormous help and advice to patients and their families.

The Bill and Melinda Gates Foundation and the globally widespread Rotary International club, along with the World Health Organization (WHO) with large-scale mass vaccinations, are extremely active and successful, but **only in the prevention area**. In this sense, we, that is to say **Polio Echo e.V**, carry on operating for the worldwide dissemination of information for our poliomyelitis friends on an honorary basis, mostly relying on donations used for information material-, printing-, electronic means- and distribution purposes.

"If you don't help yourself nobody else will"

Poliomyelitis Self-Help Organizations in Europe

• **European Polio Union:**   www.europeanpolio.eu/

• **Belgium:**
Post Polio Belgium :   www.postpolio.be

Association Francophone Polio & Post-polio (AFPPP) :
www.afppp.be

Association Belge des Paralysés (ABP) :
www.abpasbl.be
*(Please note Association Francophone Polio & Post-polio (AFPPP) &
Association Belge des Paralysés (ABP) merged with effect 1/1/2013)*

• **Czech Republic:**
Asociace Polio Ceské Republiky: www.polio.cz

• **Denmark:**
Landsforeningen af Polio-, Trafik- og
Ulykkeskadede (PTU) :   www.ptu.dk

• **Finland:**
Suomen Polioliitto Ry :   www.polioliitto.com

• **France:**
Groupe de Liaison et d'Information Post-Polio :
www.post-polio.asso.fr

• **Germany:**
Bundesverband Polio e.V. :   www.polio.sh

EIKA Aachen Polio-Forum (Associate Member) :
www.polio-forum.de

Polio Initiative Europa e.V. :   www.polio-initiative-europa.de

Polio Selbsthilfe e.V. :   www.polio-selbsthilfe.net

Polio-Echo e.V. :   www.polio-echo.eu

• **United Kingdom:**
The British Polio Fellowship :   www.britishpolio.org.uk

Polio Survivors Network :   www.poliosurvivorsnetwork.org.uk

Post-PolioUK.org: www.post-poliouk.org/

Northern Ireland Polio Fellowship: www.ni-polio.org

Scottish Post Polio Network: www.sppn.org.uk

Italy:
AIDM Onlus – Associazione Interregionale Disabili Motori Onlus :
                        www.aidmonlus.it

• **Ireland (Eire):**
Post Polio Support Group (PPSG) :
                        www.ppsg.ie

• **Niederlande** (The)
(Post)Polio Group from the VSN (Vereniging Spierziekten Nederland) :
                        www.vsn.nl

• **Norway**:
Landsforeningen for Polioskadde :
                        www.polionorway.no

• **Schweiz/Switzerland:**
Schweizerische Interessengemeinschaft für Poliomyelitis Spätfolgen
(SIPS)(Deutsch/German):
Communauté Suisse d'intérêt pour les suites tardives de la poliomyé-
lite (CISP) (Français/French):
Comunità Svizzerad'interessi dei postumi tardivi della poliomielite
(CSIP) (Italiano/Italian) :   www.polio.ch

Global Polio Eradication Initiative (Switzerland) :
                        www.polioeradication.org/

• Slovak Republic:

Polio Association of the Slovak Republic (PASR) – Asociácia polio v Slovenskej republike :

(The PASR is a specific organisation for people with polio, and family members and is part of the *Sloval Ubion* of Physically Disabled People. Its website is under construction and when live can be accessed via the link www.europeanpolio.eu/home_Members.php and under rthe subheading for Slovak Republic)

• Spain:

Asociación Afectados de Polio y Síndrome Post-Polio :

www.postpolioinfor.org

Associats de Polio I Postpolio de Catalunya (APPCAT) :

www.appcat.org

Polio Contact Organizations Worldwide

See the Post-Polio Directory of Post-Polio Health International:

http://www.post-polio.org/net/PDIR.pdf

Directories:

1) International Health Professionals & Support.

2) US Professionals & Support.

3) International & Other Useful Contacts

Firms and Organizations that Helped/Contributed
Our special thanks to:

- *Roth GmbH:*
  http://www.mobilegriffe.de/info@mobeli.de

- *Seifert Technische Orthopädie GmbH:*
  http://www.seifert-to.de/

- *Help aids – with the courtesy of Essential Aids UK:*
  http://www.essentialaids.com/kitchen-aids-feeding-aids.html

- *Some polio survivor photographs:* Rotary Club Europe

- *Information support:*

- Bundesverband Poliomyelitis e. V., Germany

- European Polio Union

- EIKA Aachen Polio-Forum, Germany

- Polio Initiative Europa e.V.

- Rotary International

- Lions Club International

- Post-Polio Health International: Directory with world-polio link addresses

- UK Patient Services Webmaster:
  http://www.patient.co.uk/health/Polio-Immunisation.html for allowing us to extract the immunization data

―――――――

Donations to: European Polio Union

EUROPEAN POLIO UNION
c/o ABP asbl
Chaussée de Gand 1434
B – 1084 Brussels

Account No: BE82 0689 0354 9468
BIC : GKCCBEBB

_____

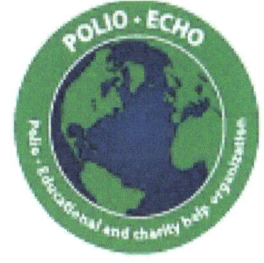

Polio-Echo e. V.

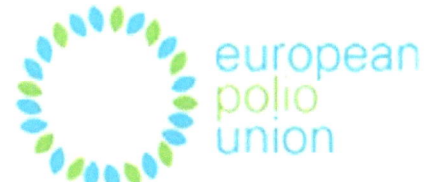

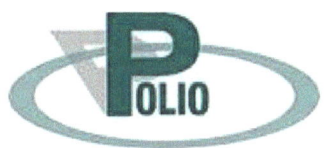

Bundesverband Poliomyelitis e. V.

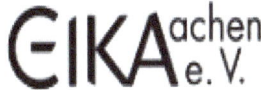

**Euregional Initiative for the late
effects of Polio - Aachen e. V.**

www.ingramcontent.com/pod-product-compliance
Lightning Source LLC
Chambersburg PA
CBHW040809200526
45159CB00022B/93